*** The Brutality of Schizophrenia***

My brother's struggle, including his writings and drawings

Maria Lazzati

For Fred

Although your time with us was too short, what you taught us will last a lifetime.

Table of Contents

The Ugly Truth about Mental Illness

People that think that they know about schizophrenia have no idea until they meet it head on, usually through a loved one.

Unless you have witnessed this horrific illness firsthand, you can't possibly imagine the fear, the frustration, the anger, the sadness, and most of all, you can't begin to understand the hopelessness you feel for your loved one.

It's an ugly fight, and the reality of it is that few ever win the battle. Schizophrenia will eat you alive and it takes your entire family with it. Each day is a new torture for these mentally ill and there is little we can do about it. The lucky ones will manage to function in this world, but they still don't fit here. Society often treats them as outcasts and many fear them. Yet they only seek comfort and the peace of not hearing the voices in their heads.

My brother, as well as all the mentally ill people of this world, was truly a special person. Sadly, many wind up on the streets simply because their families cannot handle the day to day struggles of these illnesses. Too many families have been torn apart because they did not have any support. The choices are few, you are either committed to a hospital/halfway house, you are with family or you are on the streets.

Like every other illness, education is the key to understanding. The public has to be more involved and also more tolerant.

We as a society need to start doing a better job of taking care of the mentally ill.

We need to stop ignoring the mentally ill and sweeping them under a carpet.

We need to give them all a safe place in this world, instead of giving them

one way bus fare.

This is certainly not the only occurrence of this disgusting practice, yet how many people even know that this goes on? It doesn't take a doctor to know that this isn't the answer to dealing with mental illness in our country.

Tormented and Torture

The writings shown in this book are the originals as is the art work. When I first found these legal pads filled with writings, I never thought about making them public. After reading Fred's thoughts and feelings, I wanted to share them with as many people as I could so that we all might have a better understanding of what a person with a mental illness has to live with everyday.

Tormented and tortured. Ask anyone that has a family member to describe the life of their loved one and those are usually the two words that most often are used.

Most of us get up every morning and go about our routines. We shower, dress, eat and most of us drive to work. No one tells us to do these things, we are simply living our lives and we enjoy the free will that we sometimes take for granted.

Now imagine a world where you are consumed with paranoid thoughts and voices that won't let you even take care of yourself without someone telling you to do so. If you are like me, you can't imagine your free will suddenly gone. But that is the reality of mental illness and it can happen to anyone.

An even harsher reality is that your loved one will never have the normal life that we all have. It is very difficult to accept this and when you hear of others that don't even know where their loved one is, you become grateful and thankful of what you do have.

Not only does mental illness change your loved one's lives, it changes the entire family's lives as well, and it changes things forever.

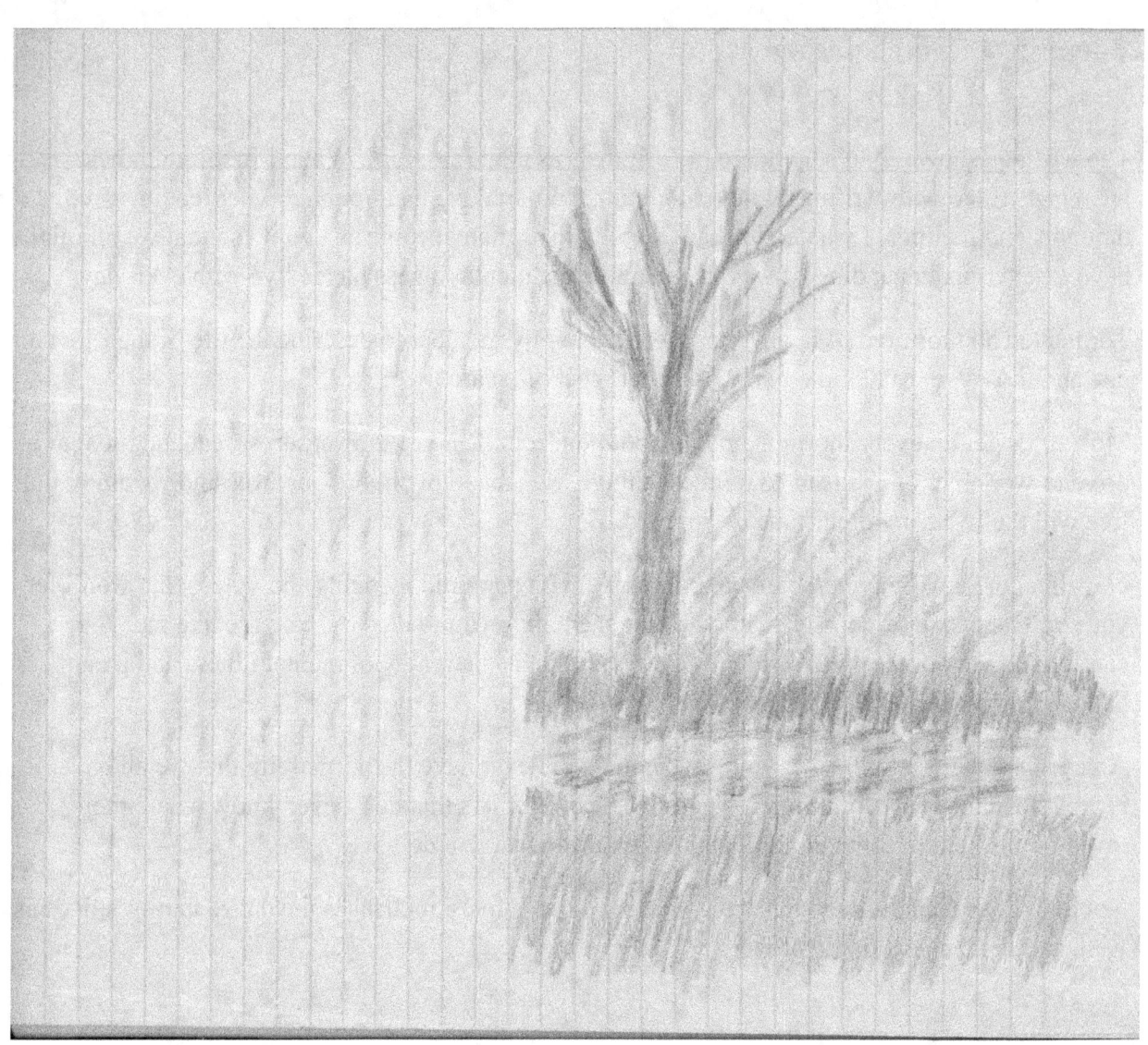

The True Brutality of Schizophrenia

Schizophrenia is a devastating illness that often destroys both the person and the family. If I sound bitter, it is because I am. My brother suffered terribly and the help available out there is almost nonexistent. For my family, not much has changed in all the years that Fred suffered.

The origins of this illness are unclear. Family history is probably the biggest and most common factor. But, some others believe it to be a virus and others believe that it might be a life event that triggers the illness.

My brother was a classic paranoid schizophrenic, yet there is no history of this illness on either side of the family. Although we all struggled along with Fred and never gave up, it wasn't until we lost him that we could finally understand the torture that he went through.

This is our family's story and we wanted to tell people that if you should have a loved one that suffers from schizophrenia, please don't ever give up. We hope that you can be lucky enough to have what we had with Fred. After many hard years of fighting this illness, we think he found some happiness, even though the symptoms never left him. In spite of this horrific illness and the tortured thoughts that robbed him of a quality life, Fred always saw the good in everything and always made the best of any situation. He was kind, sweet and giving to a fault. How he could be all that while keeping the voices in his head at bay must have truly been a struggle. But we never kidded ourselves when it came to Fred. We knew that he could not function alone in this world, as some schizophrenics are able to do.

Some of Fred 's symptoms went to extremes and they included delusions, paranoia, breaks from reality, beliefs that we tried to control his mind, government conspiracies, aggression, periods of being withdrawn, disorganized thoughts, trouble with following directions, and socialization problems. In his worst moments, there were hallucinations and constantly hearing voices. Like most schizophrenics, his physical appearance was not a priority to him, and that fact often showed through his hair and clothing.

Please note that although I may mention doctors and hospitals, this book is not from a medical viewpoint, it is about my family's struggle and Fred's torment with this mental illness. We have been through so much over the years that the timeline is a bit fuzzy for us. I broke this down into the places we've lived rather than exact dates. The events, however, are clear in our minds.

Sadly, Fred passed away suddenly on January 12, 2013 and we miss him terribly. He left a big hole in our hearts and in our lives. We will miss him for a long, long time. But we feel as though Fred was put on this Earth for a reason, and we think that reason is so that we can share his story with other families. There is always hope and you need to hang on to that. The mentally ill should not be a burden, they are special and they prove everyday how tough they are by fighting an illness that sometimes eventually wins. We need to stop hiding the mentally ill and start treating their illnesses and helping families get through this.

What many don't understand about schizophrenia is that it is an illness that affects the entire family, yet it's rarely treated as a family. It's incredibly difficult to find support and quite often, the family is isolated and left to deal with this illness on their own. I'm sure that many families were torn apart by mental illness, and ours was no different.

Although we are very grateful for having Fred for all these years, his illness was unforgiving and at many times it was downright brutal. People that do not have firsthand experience with a mentally ill loved one can't possibly imagine what we went through or what any other family goes through. It took years before Fred found medications and therapy that could help him.

The harsh reality of this is that the illness never goes away. With medication, it may be possible to function in society, but for some, it's a very unstable situation. As you will read, Fred was even able to work for a while, but in the end, the schizophrenia consumed him.

Putting Disorganized Thoughts to Paper

After Fred died, I was cleaning out a few drawers in his room and I came across a couple of legal pads that he had written and drawn on. As I read the writings and saw the pages and pages of rows of dots, it became clear to me just how tortured his mind must have been. I began to wonder if he really ever had a moment of peace. I decided to share these in this book so that you might understand how fragile a mind can be. I was once told that Fred didn't process information the same way we do, and I now believe that.

The pages shown here are all from those pads and are the originals. To correct the grammar or spelling would alter the effect and meaning. However, I did try to translate them for easier reading. The pages of dots are in the time order in which he drew these. I also have two drawings that I found within one of his books. The drawings are, unfortunately, the only ones that I have left. Fred was able to use beautiful colors and intricate designs that really make you wonder what was going through his mind. I would pass his room and see a wall full of these colorful drawings. But then they would be gone because he would throw them all out. I was always fascinated with his choice of colors as well as the designs, and I can't put into words how sorry I am that I didn't keep these drawings.

As far as his writing goes, the punctuation is terrible, and his spelling was not much better. I believe the "cogn" he uses is short for cognition. Although he sometimes put a month, day and even time, we have no idea of when he wrote these notes. Very often he would lose track of days and even years, so it's hard to say. He writes about his dots and it seems that he would draw these dots to pass the time in fifteen minute blocks. We are not sure about this "gag syndrome" that he writes about, but we imagine it's from smoking and coughing or maybe a side effect of his medication.

Here are some examples of Fred's dots on the next few pages. As you will see, he also wrote about the government not being first to see his "dot discovery on paper," and how learning that would cause "great pessimism."

These dot pages usually have a time written on them and at first I thought they were all the same, but many are different. This is why I choose to include them all and I left them in the order that he had them.

Rough Seas

Thursday September 25

Rough seas tonight, seems trouble is forthcoming. I can feel the bouncing. My fears lie within the basic four walls of the house. Everywhere I go, I should do something.

There is a fear that can't be dealt with, the fear of an unknown, not dangerous destiny.

Daily Struggles of a Mental Illness

Our family felt that we had to get this story out, especially for those that are going through the same day to day struggle as we did. It was nothing compared to the battles that Fred had to face each and every day. But, Fred will live on in all of us, and we will always hope and pray that things change for the families of the mentally ill and that help isn't just for the wealthy or the ones that live on the streets. That was always very frustrating for us. We were always told that if Fred had been homeless, there would be all kinds of help available. The system needs work and thanks to the dedicated people we have met along the way, there's always the hope that change is near.

Even though Fred was on disability and it helped with the bills, it rarely covered his expenses. I'm sure other families in our situation will agree that financial help just doesn't exist. Most months, we barely got by. We managed, but there should be some financial help available to the families that offer our loved ones a warm and safe place to live, hot meals every day, clothing, medication, and other expenses that we dealt with. Fred never knew that we struggled with these expenses and we didn't want him to worry. Even support groups are hard to come by.

We live in a great country that often helps other nations and countries with their burdens, yet they turn their backs on their own people that need help the most. It seems as though every time a politician needs to make a budget cut, it is often taken from the seniors or the mentally ill. Sadly, until a politician has a mentally ill child or loved one with this horrible illness and is emotionally and financially drained, things will probably never change. That is just another reality of mental illness and families like mine known this all too well.

Even after Fred passed away, we thought there might be something out there to help us with his final expenses. We were wrong. We couldn't even find help with his funeral. The worst part about this is that all we keep hearing is that if Fred was homeless, everything would have been paid for. That's the part that I find difficult. We have a system that tells us that you are better off living on the streets rather than with a loving family. There is something very wrong with this system.

I am not suggesting that the state support my family and pay all the bills, but there should be something in place to help the families that struggle. Taking care of Fred was almost a full time job in itself and we had a lot of expenses. When his doctor sent Fred for tests a few years ago, we had to pay for all the medical bills that weren't covered by Medicare. No matter what the cost, I would have done anything it took to keep my brother safe with me.

There has to be some better financial support in place for those that cannot afford the care that the mentally ill require. My parents literally went broke trying to keep Fred in the better psychiatric facilities that only offer care to those that can pay. As a parent, you have no regrets or second thoughts about doing this, but in the end, it probably didn't matter much as far as his illness goes. What does matter is finding the right medication and the right team of support for these mentally ill patients and their families. Sadly, even with the best treatments, some are still lost forever. There were times that we felt that way about Fred, but then he would get better for a while.

You don't have to be a doctor to sense the torture or struggles that Fred faced. Just reading his notes left me wondering how he ever functioned at all. That's why it was so important to my family that we share what we had with Fred, including the good days and more important, the bad days. Seeing Fred's original writings are far more effective that just writing about them. We also printed the paged of dots because they meant something to Fred, yet we will never understand what they represented in his mind. After reading the following, it's hard to imagine feeling the way Fred describes. It's harder to imagine the torment that he suffered but it's clear from his writings that he struggled more than we thought.

Dots and Government Conspiracy

Entry

Even if the government was aware of my cognition, it would go to them second or third, first consulting with the doctors, then the scientists. So the government would really be third in the chain, not first. I guess I had it in the reverse.

Anyway, with my new dot on paper discovery, this is a time for great pessimism.

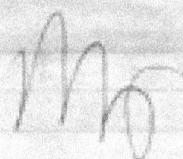

12:05

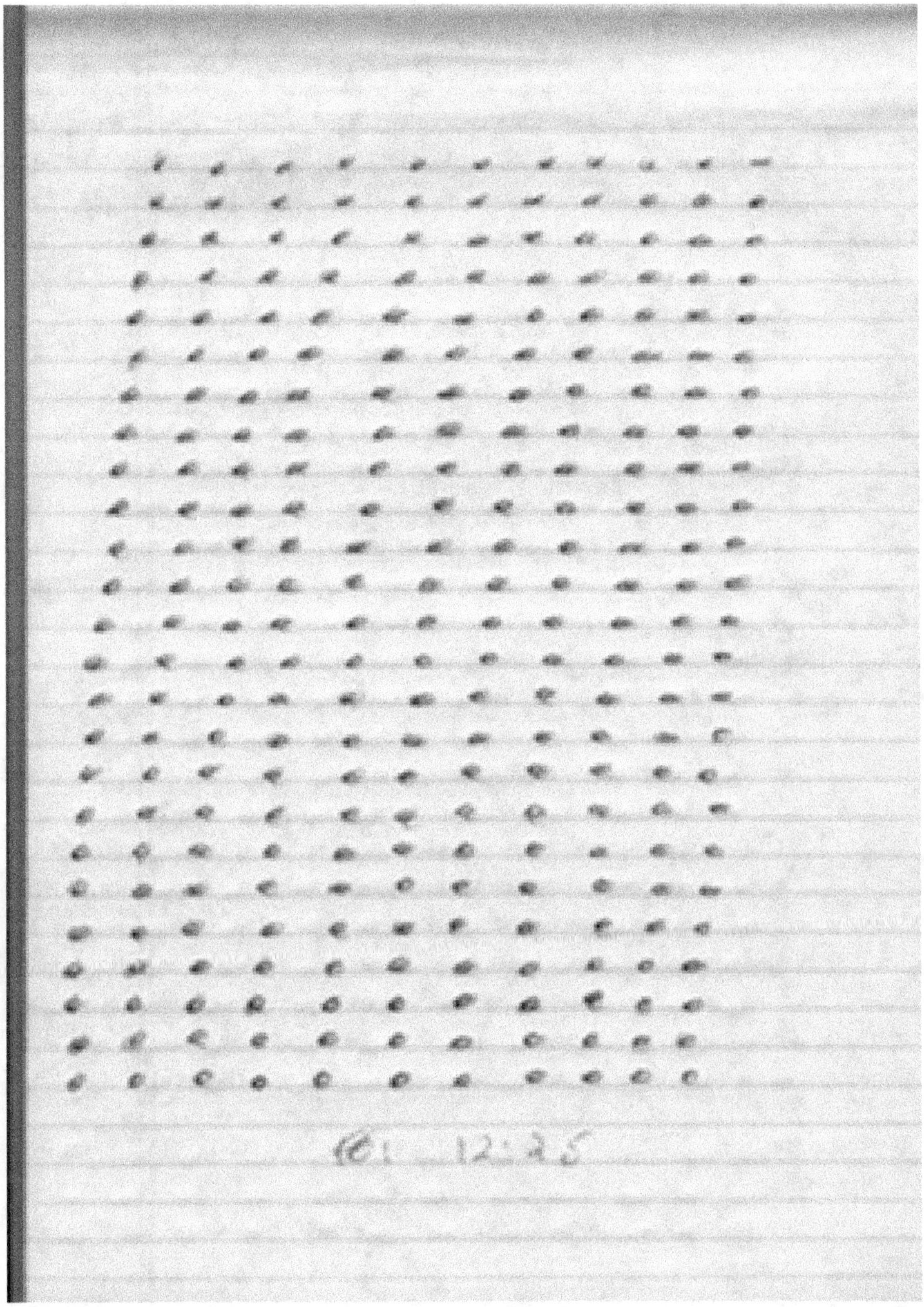
12:25

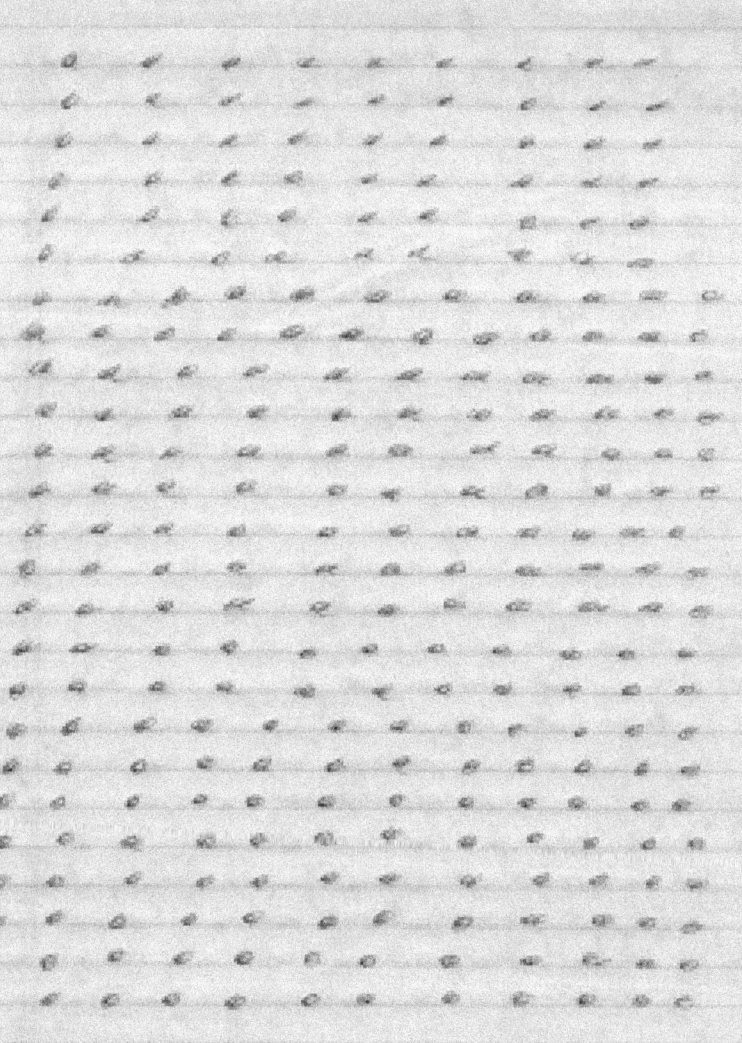

12145

15.15

The Stigma of Being Mentally Ill

Unfortunately, the mentally ill are usually swept under a rug and hidden from view. Every time a mentally ill person makes the news, it is quickly made to look as though all mentally ill people are violent and aggressive. Ignorance takes control and opinions fly. Some folks believe that all mentally ill people should just be locked up. Others think there should be a database not unlike what we have for child abusers and predators. A lot of people mistakenly believe that the mentally ill are violent. Actually, I have read many times that the mentally ill are in fact more likely to be victims of crime, not the aggressor. The suicide rate is much higher with a schizophrenic, as well.

Too many times we have watched the news and listened to the reports of yet another mentally ill person shooting, stabbing or killing those around him or her. But what you will likely never hear is the story behind this person and that he or she probably never received medical treatment and in place of that treatment, turned to drugs or alcohol to stop the symptoms. This is what people should be aware of and should understand. Left to itself, a mental illness will only get worse. We all know horrific ending that some episodes could take. Most mentally ill people are just scared and I know in Fred's case, he just wanted the voices to stop. It's incredibly difficult to explain to friends and even other family members understand the brutality of schizophrenia. Every day was a struggle for Fred and there was little that we could do to help him. Although he appeared to be happy, as you will read in his notes, he was the most tortured soul that I ever knew, and I am sorry that I couldn't do more for him.

Fred was not violent, but if you saw him, you might cross the street because he didn't look like us. His hair was a little wild and his clothes were usually disheveled. He was often not paying attention to his surroundings and seemed to be wandering aimlessly. You might even think he was homeless. But if you spoke with him or greeted him, he would be happy to converse with you and you would find him to be friendly and cheerful.

His appearance was just the nature of his mental illness, so we took what we could get and were happy to have him.

Fred was constantly haunted by these voices and some days must have been such a fight for him. Yet he never complained or told us how bad things were. In fact, Fred had the most amazing ability to take the worse possible situation and find some good in it. That was Fred's gift and it is something that I miss every single day.

Although we always loved Fred, it took his passing to make us realize just how lucky and blessed we were to even have had him in our lives. It is how I find the motivation to educate as many people as I can as to the realities of mental illness.

Fact is, having schizophrenia means that it won't always have a happy ending. Sadly, many of the mentally ill will wind up homeless and living on the streets. If you read the story at the beginning, you now know that some states routinely ship these homeless people to other locations. I have read that some hospitals will treat the mentally ill and when they are capable of traveling, they will ship them to another destination, often without money or medication. This is not the exception- this is fast becoming the rule.

Do I have a solution? No, but I do know that this is not even humane, let alone moral. Again, I do believe that if more help and education is available for the families, maybe some of the mentally ill can have a chance of staying with them. It is absolutely overwhelming trying to deal with a loved one with mental illness. I don't claim to have the answers, but I do know from living with Fred for many years that it is possible to give them a home where they feel safe and non-threatened.

The Weeks Mornings

weeks

The ~~weeks~~ (mornings)

monDay I'LL wake up,
Do the Same thing I've
Been Doing For 2 years
TuesDay I'LL wake up, and
Do the same Thing I've
Been Doing For 2 years
weDnsDay I'LL wake up
and Do the Same thing I've
Been Doing For 2 years
ThursDay I'LL wake up and
Do the Same thing I've
Been Doing For 2 years
FriDay I'LL wake up and
Do the Same thing I've
Done For 2 years
SaturDay I wake up and
Do the Same thing I've
Done For 2 years
SunDay I'LL wake up and
Do the same thing I've
Done For 2 years
I Do I've Done the Same
thing in the morning For
2 years

7:00

7:25

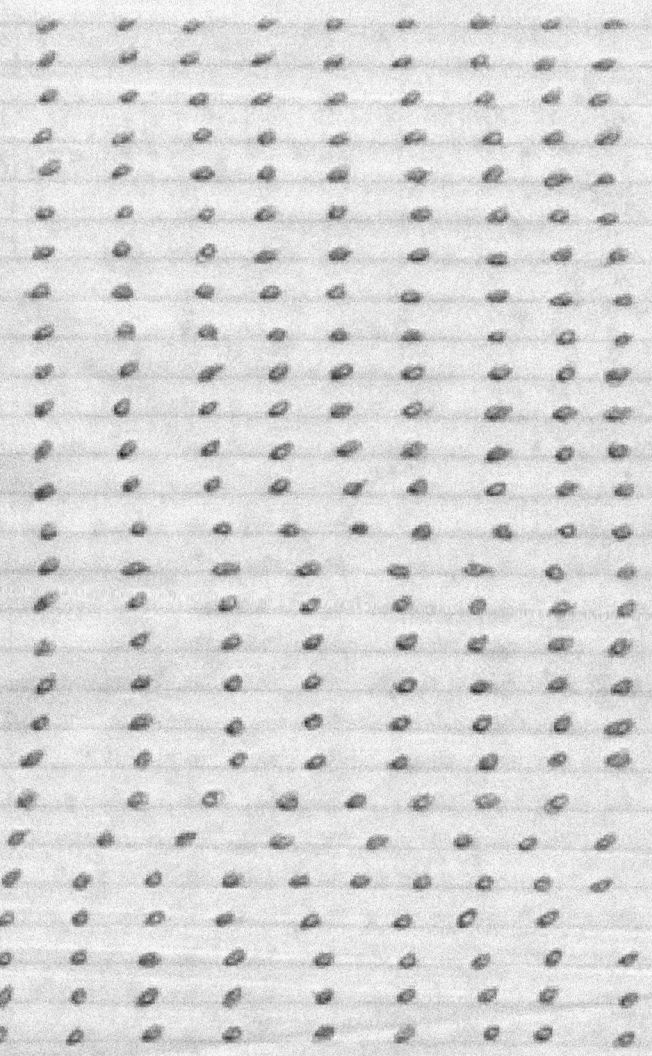

8 | 16

You Just Don't Think About Mental Illness

My brothers and I grew up in Long Island and later moved to the northern NJ area. Fred had been a normal kid. We were lucky to have two wonderful and loving parents. My father was a good man and worked hard to give us everything. My mother stayed home and worked just as hard to give us a beautiful home. I always remembered Fred as being an awesome athlete. It seemed like he excelled at every sport that he played.

I can't put a date on the first time that we suspected a problem with Fred, in fact, I was in my early teens and Fred was probably about 17 years old, so about 40 years ago. That's the nature of mental illness. Sometimes it comes suddenly and out of the blue. One day everything is fine and the next day you realize that your life will never be the same again. But then one day you look back and you realize all the signs were there, you just didn't know what they were.

I know that I remember that Fred's behavior had changed sometime in high school- probably his senior year and that would be in the mid to late 70's. He seemed to be angry all the time and would go and come at home as he pleased. We suspected drugs, and we knew he did in fact use whatever he could buy at school or on the streets. Fred and I went to the same school and some of my friends were the sisters of his friends, so I had a good idea of what was going on. Many people I knew experimented with some of these drugs, mostly amphetamines, pot and lots of alcohol. Watching Fred was enough to scare me from experimenting with anything.

When someone you know and love begins to slowly change before your eyes, no one thinks, "Hmmm, he must be mentally ill." You think drugs, you think alcohol you think of any excuse but mental illness. In Fred's case, the drug part was true. My friends at school would tell me that Fred was indeed pan handling for drugs on the streets at night. They laughed and told me how me funny he was while trying to sell forks that he had taken from our home. My heart would sink when I heard these stories. I didn't have a clue about mental illness, but still I felt truly sorry for Fred. These people laughing had no clue what was going on, and we didn't either. But I just know that something was very wrong.

Eventually, he would come home and go to bed and get up and go to school the next morning. As far as school went, Fred was pretty average. He was a good looking guy and always had a girlfriend. But now he was using drugs and his behavior was getting more aggressive towards us.

I remember one day in his senior year, Fred came home and told us to take him to a hospital because he was sick. He thought he had mono, but it was actually Hepatitis A. I remember how yellow his eyes were and since it was infectious, we had to get vaccinated. Of course we suspected it was from the drug use, but the Board of Health actually traced it back to a restaurant where he had eaten shellfish. Fred was quarantined in the hospital and only my parents were allowed to see him. Although he made a full recovery, he was not permitted to return to school and was tutored for the remainder of the school year.

After high school, Fred tried a community college, but it didn't last long. My father worked in the textile business and Fred started working for him loading trucks and doing odd jobs. Again, he was okay for a while, but nothing could keep this illness from coming back. He would have a few other jobs when he was young, but they would eventually end when his illness became too much to fight.

Fred became withdrawn and stayed in his room most of the time. When he became agitated, my father would talk to him and calm him down. When I look back, I am truly amazed at the effect that my father had on Fred. My parents made it their life's mission to learn as much about schizophrenia as they possibly could. They would speak with doctors, attend lectures, they would read anything on the subject and my father would talk for hours with Fred and almost always would get him back to a calm state.

Tomorrow

Sept 20 Thurs
Tommorrow

Tommorrow I will get
up to follow the same
Routine gag in the morning
get wake up get up
& smoke have coffee
and sit Down try to fight
this cogni thing and
my gag syndrome will
come on ~~strikethrough~~ seems
to be a big factor in my
anger and Paranoic ~~strikethrough~~
tendencies I won't change
the ~~First~~ first half
a hour of my morning
IF I DiD somthing would
have to change its
sad Just have coffee
standing up then when
my gag syndrome starts
up Do Exercises or
Somthing

Living with the Symptoms

The hardest part of this illness is the fact that it is so unpredictable. One day Fred would be fine, the next he would be agitated and sullen. Some days he could not do enough for us, other days we wouldn't be able to get him to even take a bag of trash out. Some days his paranoia would be extreme and he would complain about neighbors looking at him funny or tell us how they were annoyed that he was walking and sometimes he would tell us that some shirts/belongings were missing from his room. In his worst moments, he believed he was being poisoned and threw all his food out.

Sometimes, Fred would become sullen and not speak to us. Other times, he might laugh to himself to a point where it was uncomfortable for us to witness. If he noticed us, he would explain that he had just thought of something funny, but we knew it was just another part the illness. At one point, he talked of sometimes hearing voices, but he said he knew that were only in his mind and he could keep them at bay.

We wanted Fred to be normal so badly that we often hid behind denial. That's the problem with schizophrenia. It's not until you look back that you realize that something had changed.

Most families caring for a schizophrenic will agree that it is a very unpredictable illness. You could be outgoing, agreeable, happy, talkative, helpful, and very lucid today, and tomorrow you could be withdrawn, angry, and moody. Over time, we began to recognize his moods and avoided asking him things that might upset him or cause him to pace. Sometimes we had to deal head on with an issue, maybe his appearance or trying to get him to change his clothes. It would sometimes end with him telling us to call his doctor and tell him about it. He would say, "I don't see anything wrong with what I'm wearing, but if you want, call my doctor and tell him that you don't like what I'm wearing," or "Just because you don't like what I'm wearing doesn't mean that I should have to change. Maybe I don't like what you're wearing, would you go change?" Conversations like this were common and at times, very frustrating.

We tried to keep Fred busy with chores and productive things just so he wouldn't sit up in his room all day. He seemed to enjoy the responsibility of having us depend on him. I would ask him to watch over our mother while I was at work and he would help her around the house.

When Fred was worried about something, he would pace all day and all night. He would pace in the house and he would pace outside. He wouldn't eat and he would smoke like a chimney and drink coffee nonstop. His agitation would be obvious and we always tried to make a bad situation hopeful so that Fred would calm down.

Then there were times when Fred would become agitated for reasons unknown to us. Looking back, we wonder if Fred was feeling ill or struggling with another symptom of his schizophrenia. He went every two weeks for his injection of Risperdal, and sometimes when he was in the second week, he would show more symptoms. It was almost as if the medication wore off too soon. After his injection, he would be okay for a while.

Sadly, there were times when Fred wouldn't walk into a room if someone was already there. If I was in the kitchen cooking, Fred might fill a cup with water for coffee, then just set it down and walk away. I would tell him to come back but he would say, "No, that's okay. I'll wait until you're done."

It was the same if you walked into a room where Fred was. If he was sitting in the den and you came in, he'd grab his cup and cigarettes and go up to his room. We all felt bad about that, but it was typical Fred and no matter how many times we told him not to leave, he would.

We don't know if that was a part of the paranoia or just another symptom of his illness. Some days he might come down and ask us how we were doing and talk with us for a while. Some days he would be so intensely engrossed in his thoughts that he wouldn't even hear us talking.

Like I said, some days you have to just accept what you have and hope that tomorrow is a little better.

101:10

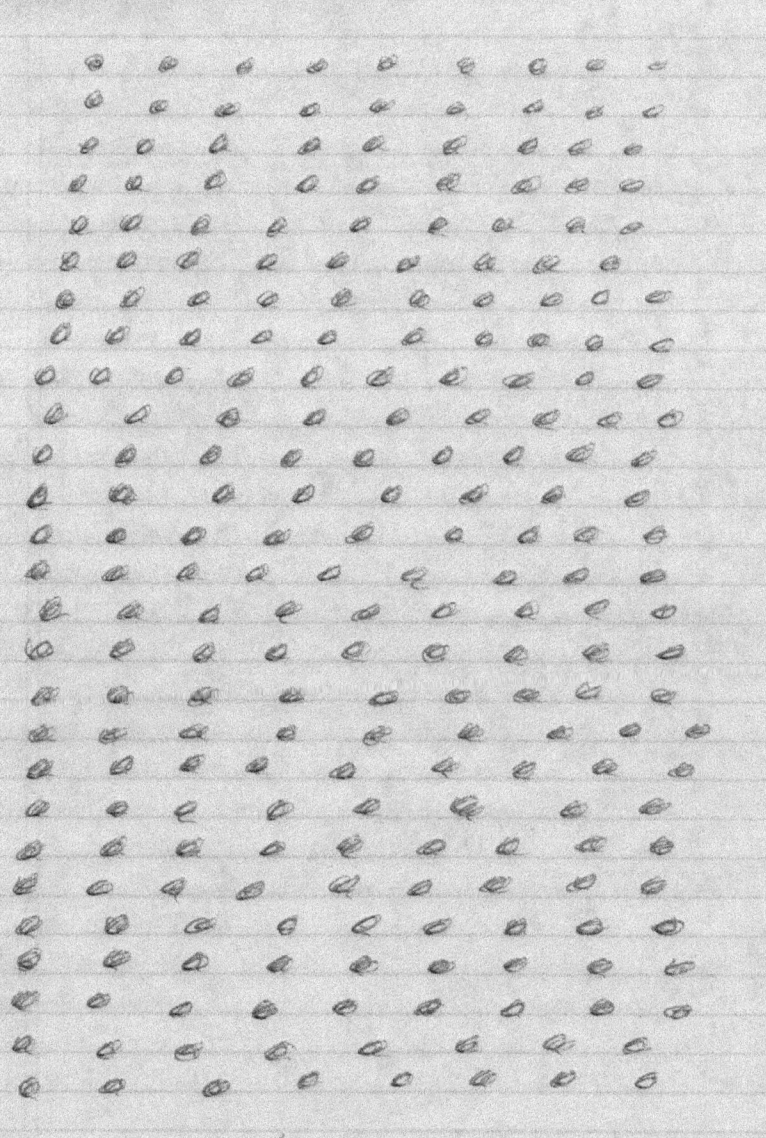

10:30

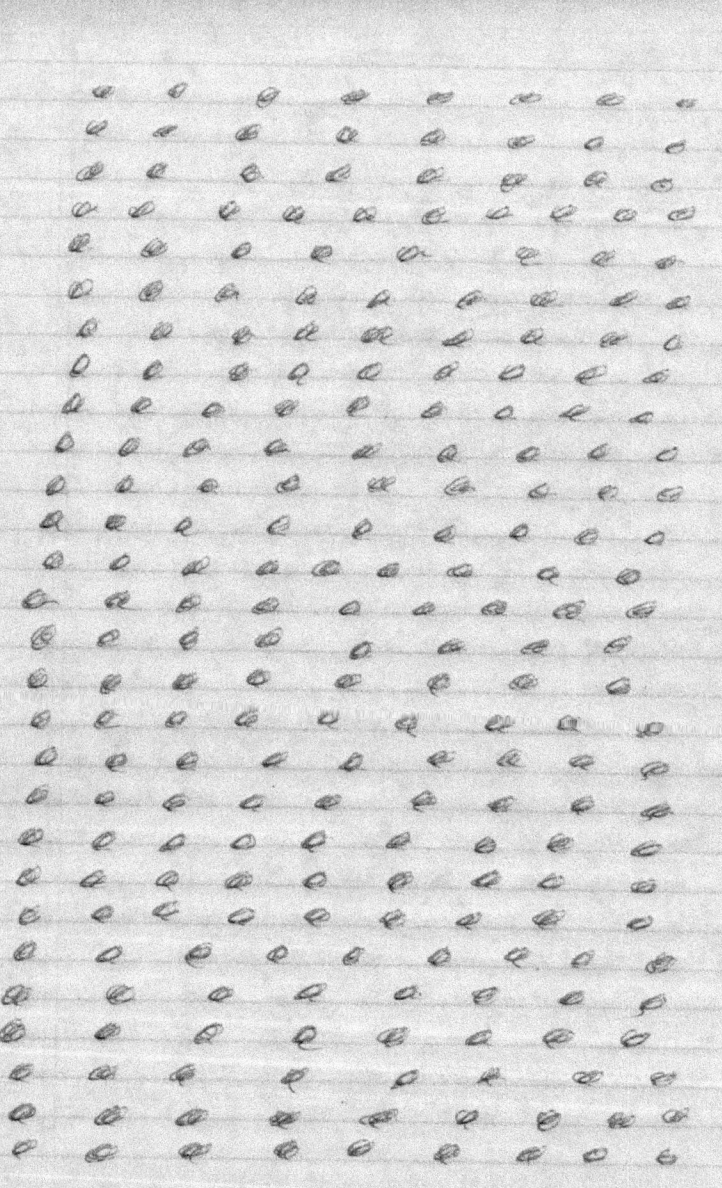

10150

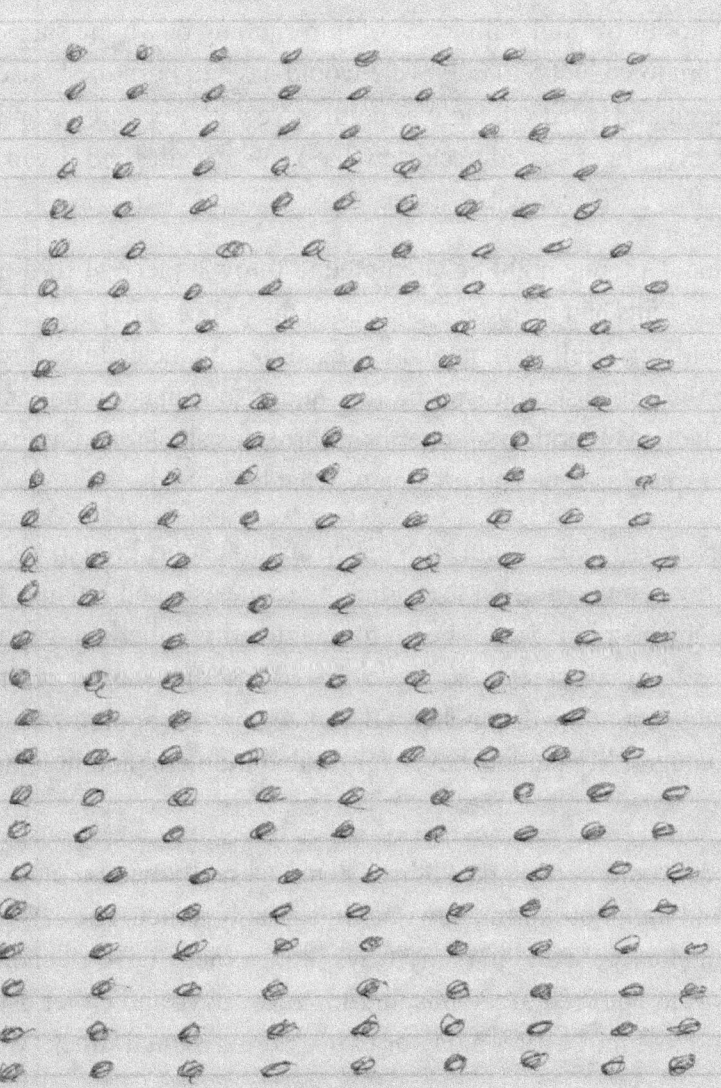

11:10

The Long Road for Families

One of my earliest memories of Fred's illness is of him running down the stairs and telling my parents that God told him to collect $20,000 or he would have to burn the house down. I remember being confused and petrified. He was combative with my parents and I remember that when I looked into his eyes, I got scared because what I saw wasn't Fred. Even at my young age, I knew at that moment that Fred was not in there.

Shortly after the first incident, one night he attempted to throw a piece of furniture through his bedroom window. My parents had no choice but to call the police. They now knew that Fred's anger and agitation could very well be a mental issue, so they requested that Fred be brought to a hospital. They were in the police station waiting for a judge to sign commitment papers so that Fred could be sent for help. My mother said her heart broke as she looked at Fred just sitting in a jail cell staring out into space as if he had no idea of what happened.

An officer asked a dispatcher to contact an ambulance and transport Fred to the hospital. The dispatcher, in front of my parents, gets on the radio and requests an ambulance to pick up "some wacko" and get him to the hospital. I can't begin to imagine my father's anger and hurt at hearing the dispatcher refer to his son as "some wacko." My father started yelling at everyone and later he told the judge about the dispatcher. Of course, they all apologized, but obviously only because they got caught. My parents never forgot that moment, and how heartbroken they were to hear it.

From that moment, Fred would now be part of a system that really had no clue as to how to deal with the mentally ill, and I am not faulting anyone, it is simply a fact. The 1970's and even the 80's were hard on the mentally ill, and in many ways, things today haven't changed much. The answer society gave was to put Fred in the hospital for a few days and either drug him 24 hours a day or just hold him and let him go after a day or two, as if his mental illness would go away like the flu.

As his behavior worsened, he would disappear for days at a time. He would sometimes come home and threaten us. His agitation was escalating, but we lived in a society that required Fred to hurt someone or himself before he could be arrested or committed. We sometimes didn't know if it was worse when he was home or when he wasn't. He was becoming increasingly paranoid and he would accuse us of controlling his thoughts and mind. This would make him more aggressive.

In all the years with battling mental illness, although Fred was threatening and acting aggressively, he never once hurt any of us nor was he ever destructive, except for the night he tried to shove furniture out his window. The problem is that at the time, we didn't know that he would not hurt anyone, and we believed that he was very capable of hurting someone. That made him extremely scary to me. I went from feeling sorry for him to trying to block him out of my life. He became a monster in my eyes, and I am ashamed to say that I avoided him at all costs and fought with my parents because I felt that they should just throw him out. He disrupted my childhood, he disrupted my time with my parents, he disrupted my life and I wanted it to end.

Our house was the one where our friends would come and hang out. We slowly stopped inviting friends over out of fear of Fred's unpredictable behavior. And my anger at Fred would worsen and I would also be angry with my parents for letting our family fall apart.

I remember coming home from school one day and when I opened the door, Fred was sitting on the steps in our hallway and I thought he was flipping through a family photo album, but then I realized that he had a red marker in his hands and he was placing an "x" on the faces of my parents in the photos. I will never forget the fear that I felt when he stopped and looked up at me and said "I'll give you ten seconds to get out of the house." I just backtracked out the door and waited in my car for my parents to come back. To this day I remember believing that Fred was possessed, because what I saw that day was not him.

That's the sad part about schizophrenia. It rips families apart because the illness has so many unknowns and it totally unpredictable. I look back now and I am absolutely stunned and awed at the love my parents had for us. They refused to let him go, they refused to believe that he couldn't be helped, they refused to believe that he needed to live in some institution.

Whenever we questioned my parents and their decision to help Fred, they would say that this illness was no different than having a child with cancer, and no parent would ever walk away from trying to save that child, no matter what the cost.

My parents had just started their long but dedicated journey down a road that would include conflicting psychiatric opinions, more police, heartbreak, endless frustration and many nights either of lying awake wondering where Fred was or driving around looking for him. My parents did that a lot. They would go out at night and just drive around looking for Fred. This became a routine for them, and I now can't imagine how they dealt with all this.

I remember times when the hospital or halfway house where Fred was staying would call and ask us if Fred was home. Of course, my parents would freak out because he was supposed to be there. How Fred was able to just wander away has always puzzled us. But, like so many other nights, my parents would get in the car and search for Fred. My father was still working at the time, so after working a full day, this is what he came home to. My parents never gave a second thought to getting out of bed, getting dressed and going out looking for Fred for half the night.

Differing Medical Opinions

During the first few years when Fred's schizophrenia was manifesting and taking control of his life, he had been taken to a hospital several times for observation and treatment. It was during these times that my parents were given conflicting opinions from doctors and psychiatrists.

One doctor thought Fred was perfectly fine and just having a rough patch of some sort. Another blamed my parents for the illness and said Fred was ok but they needed help. Yet another said Fred needed to be institutionalized and could never be a part of our family. Sometimes the hospitals would keep Fred for a few days, sometimes weeks. Some hospitals were better than others, and some tried to help Fred with therapy and medication. But some just drugged him 24 hours a day. It if all sounds hit or miss, that's exactly how I remember it.

He would eventually wind up being committed in Greystone for a while. Doctors were scarce and their idea of help was sedation. I remember that more than once, Fred would manage to walk away and he would show up at our home. We would let him in and call my father at work. He would come home and try to talk Fred into going back. Meanwhile, we would sit in fear and pray he didn't do anything. The point is, even when Fred was in a hospital, we lived in fear that he would show up. At the time, Greystone was nothing more than a warehouse, and it was a hopeless choice. My father wouldn't even let me visit Fred there, it was that bad. Again, this was back quite a few years, so hopefully, things have since changed.

This would become a standard way of life for us. Fred would be okay for a while, then his illness would take over and we would either call the police or try to talk him into going to the hospital. Sometimes, Fred would wander off for days, even weeks. There were gaps when we had no idea where he was or if he was even okay. My parents would spend hours driving around looking for him. Eventually, he would show up again.

Waiting for the Sun

Entry   4:20 thurs)
                    sept 25
    waiting For the sun (song)
or my Dot ~~key~~ technique
to Form ~~yo~~ 2 Days ago
was   a Damaging hurricane.
today all is calm its
Exciting and optimism at
its Best But Still there
is to many ~~fift~~ Fifteen
minute gaps Ive Done
Somthing similar to this
Before it worked Better
than I know or knew
this one Seems to have
Done the same its
~~4:0~~ 4:~~30~~25   Voices sound
vengful and Bitter and
Direct Hateful Bed person
Furious in a Disagreeable
and unforgiving and Dangerous
way Parinoia Slight mood
over Enthusiastic and
Anxious, Expectant

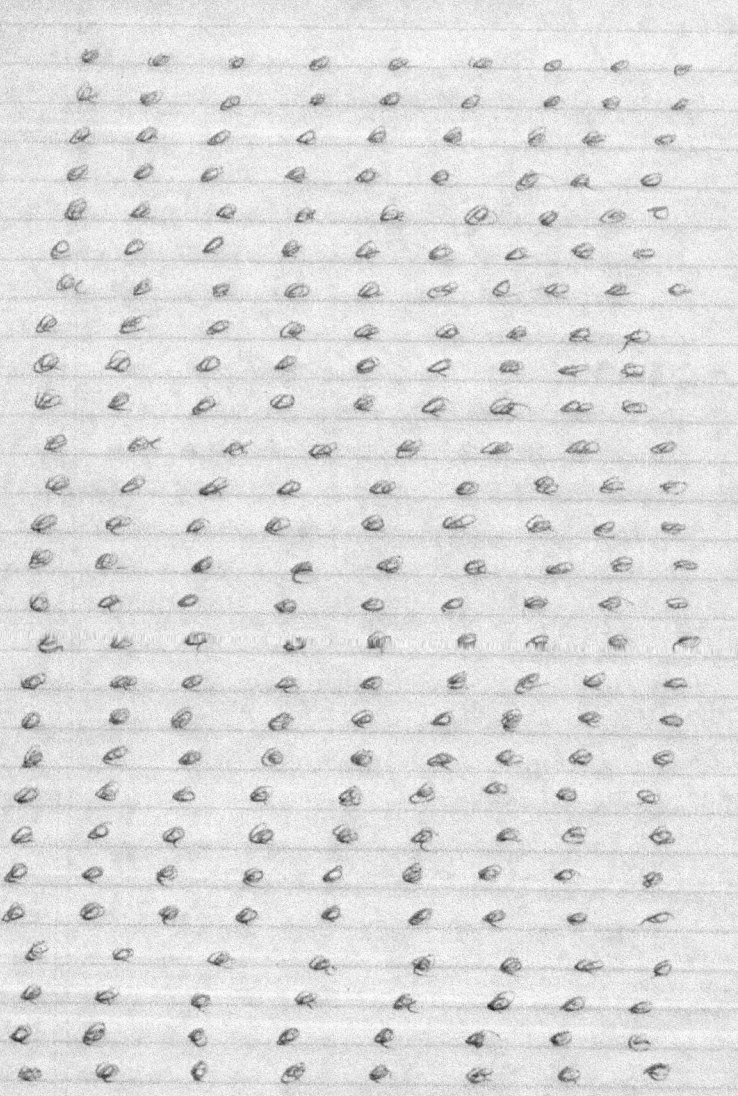

211

2:35

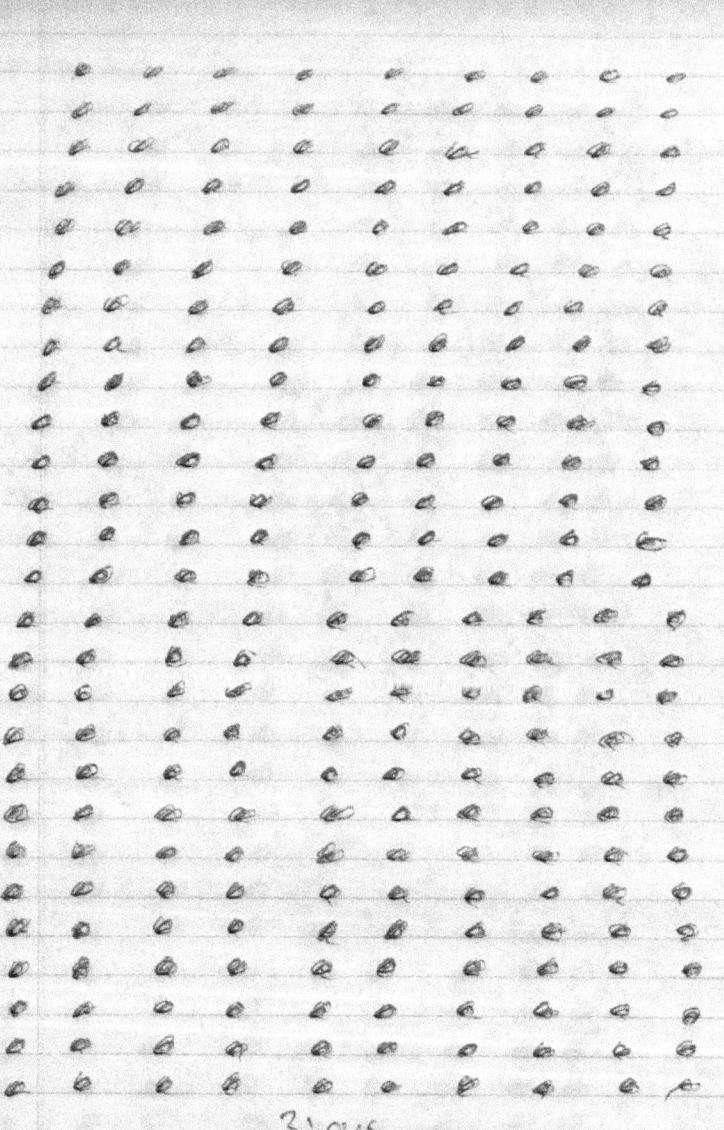

3:00

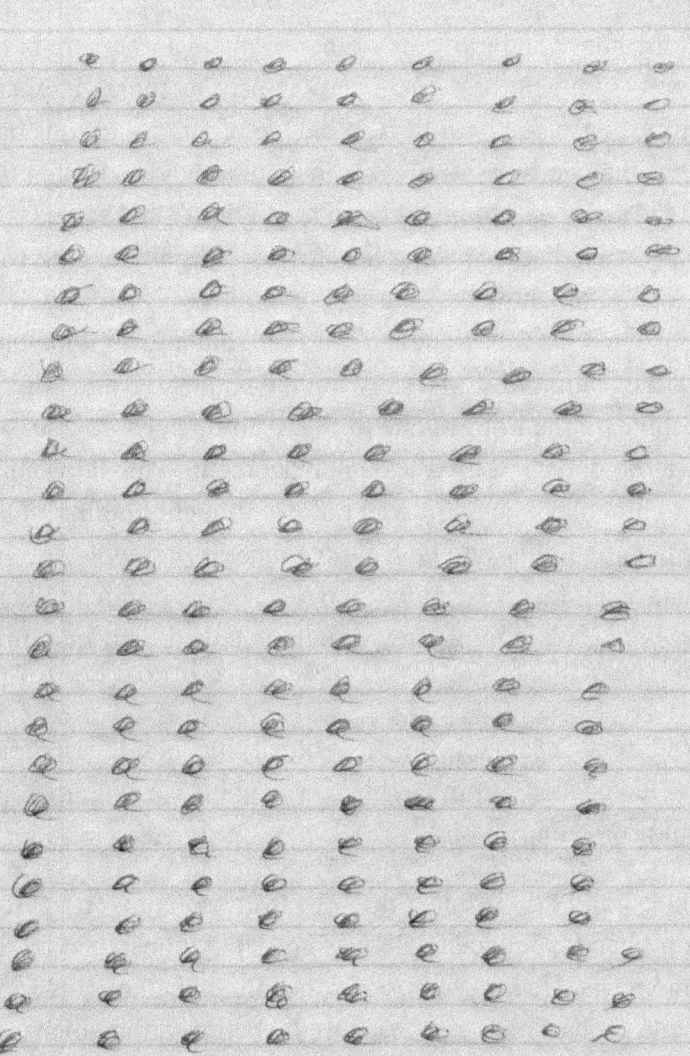

3110

It Gets Worse before it Gets Better

My parents decided to sell the house and move, my other brothers and I were in college or moved out and the house was too much for them. Once my parents found another house, they moved right away and left the house empty until it sold. One night, my friends had gone to the house to pick up some things that we were storing for them and they said when they walked in, Fred came barreling down the stairs screaming at them to get out. What scared them more was the smell of gas, Fred had a terrible habit of using the stove as a lighter and he would leave the gas on if the pilot light was out. Somehow they were able to turn off the gas before they left and then they called me. Of course my parents went and got Fred, but a few nights later, my parents received a call from the frantic realtor who was showing the house. He said when he went upstairs, he saw a man sleeping on the floor in one of the bedrooms. Of course, we immediately knew that it was Fred. It was obvious that Fred had an attachment to the house that kept bringing him back. It didn't matter to him that we had moved out. He thought nothing of that fact. He didn't care that there were not any lights, and he had no concerns of people coming in. We didn't know how many days he had spent there. By now my parents were frantic at the thought of the new owners moving in and Fred showing up. They somehow talked Fred into moving near them and found him an apartment a few blocks away.

As you will read in Fred's writings, change is the most horrifying and devastating event and it could easily paralyze him. Fred needed routine in his world and if we even mentioned change of any kind, his agitation would come on full blast.

I look back at the Fred's illness and I realize that this was the absolute worst part of it. Moving was a change that he couldn't handle or accept. He was now fully consumed by this illness and there were no more lucid moments. He accused us of controlling his thoughts and his mind. He tied white sweat socks around each of his wrists because he believed that aliens wanted him to slit his wrists with a cigarette lighter. He began to wear a heavy dirty winter coat in the middle of summer. His hair was long and so filthy that it was matted and wild. He would go into the store across the street, buy some food and when he got back to his apartment, he would throw it away. He believed all the food was poisoned. My parents would stop in to clean and check on him and they said the garbage can was full of unopened packaged food, even cans. Neighbors were afraid of him and complained. He had no clue of time, didn't know the day of the week or even the year. I believed that Fred was gone for good and yet I struggled with the ignorance of his illness.

I would often turn my ignorance into anger at Fred for being ill. Somehow, I wanted to believe that Fred could control this and I wanted him to stop being sick.

Whenever they visited, my parents would hang out for a while, but Fred would be locked in his bedroom and many times didn't even know that they were there. Sometimes he would come out and tell them to leave. I was at the apartment one day with my parents and Fred was having a very bad day. He was very agitated and pacing all over, smoking one cigarette after another. My father had been in touch with a doctor who said he would come over and evaluate Fred, and he did. He said Fred needed to be hospitalized and treatment would be lengthy. The problem was that we could not force or commit him, nor could we get the medication that would help him. This frustration was a constant part of our lives and led to many fights within our family. We always felt like our hands were tied and we couldn't do anything for Fred, It was almost hopeless.

If Fred wasn't in the apartment, they would wait for him or go looking. Sometimes they would find him walking aimlessly around the neighborhood. I can't begin to imagine the heartache of watching your child being eaten alive by an illness that robs the mind of any chance at normalcy. Whenever I saw Fred walking around with those socks tied around his wrists and that matted hair, it broke my heart, so I can't even pretend to know the pain that my parents felt.

One night Fred got picked for pan handling and when my parents went to pick him up, a policeman said to my brother, "This is a nice town and we don't want people like you here, so stay away." This was the ignorance that we put up with, and many probably still do. Mental illness makes people uncomfortable. There are a few links at the end of this book of instances where these mentally ill are picked up on the street, treated at a hospital then given bus fare out of town. When society stops looking at the mentally ill as burdens and instead finds them help, we will all be better off. Ignoring it won'

My mother still reminds me that she and my father would never, ever abandon Fred, no matter how bad things got. "You don't abandon your child because they're sick," is what she tells us. My parents always promised each other that they would never give up on Fred, and they never did. As I got older, and after my father passed away, I started to get much more involved in Fred's care. I also vowed never to leave Fred behind or stop taking care of him.

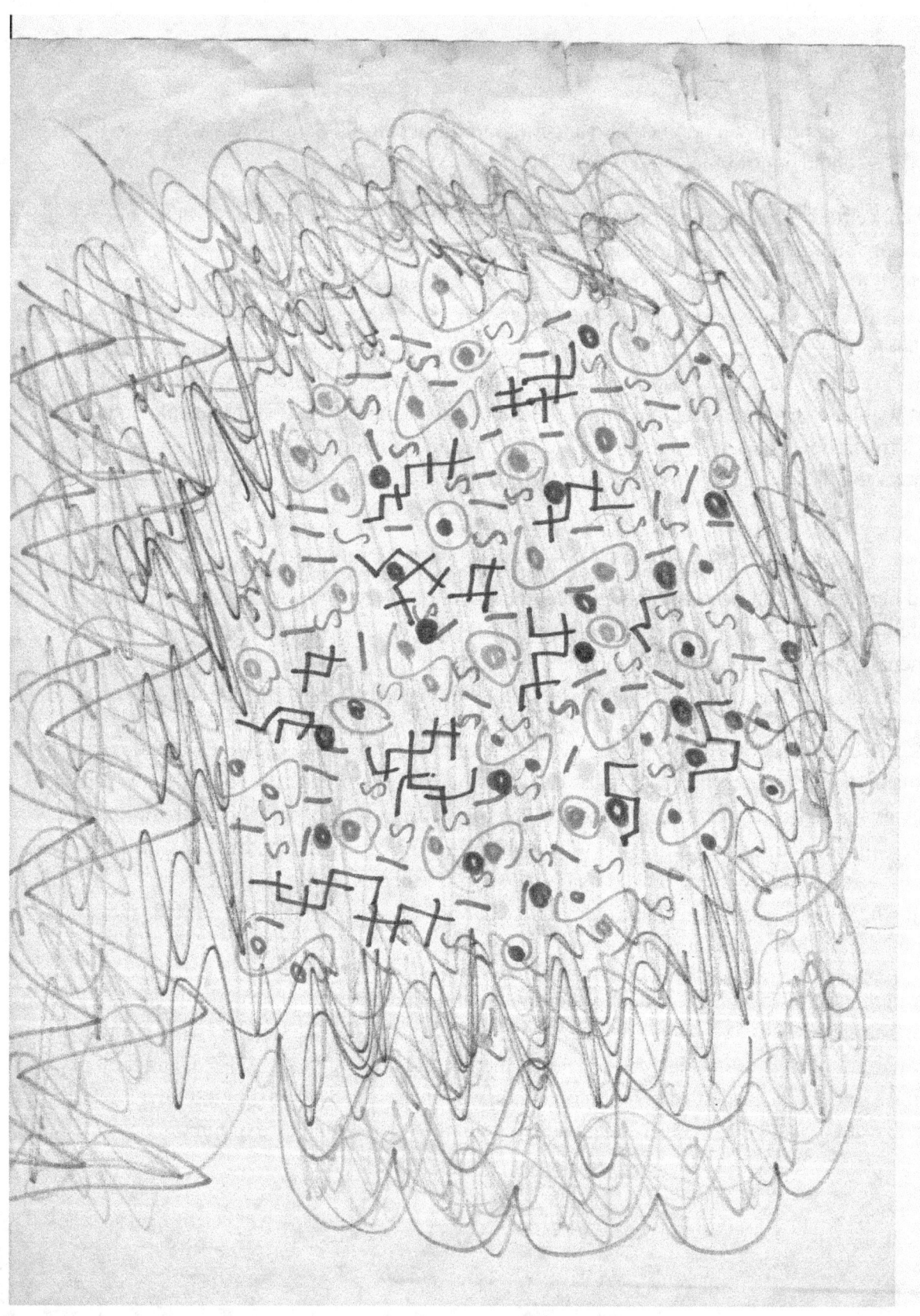

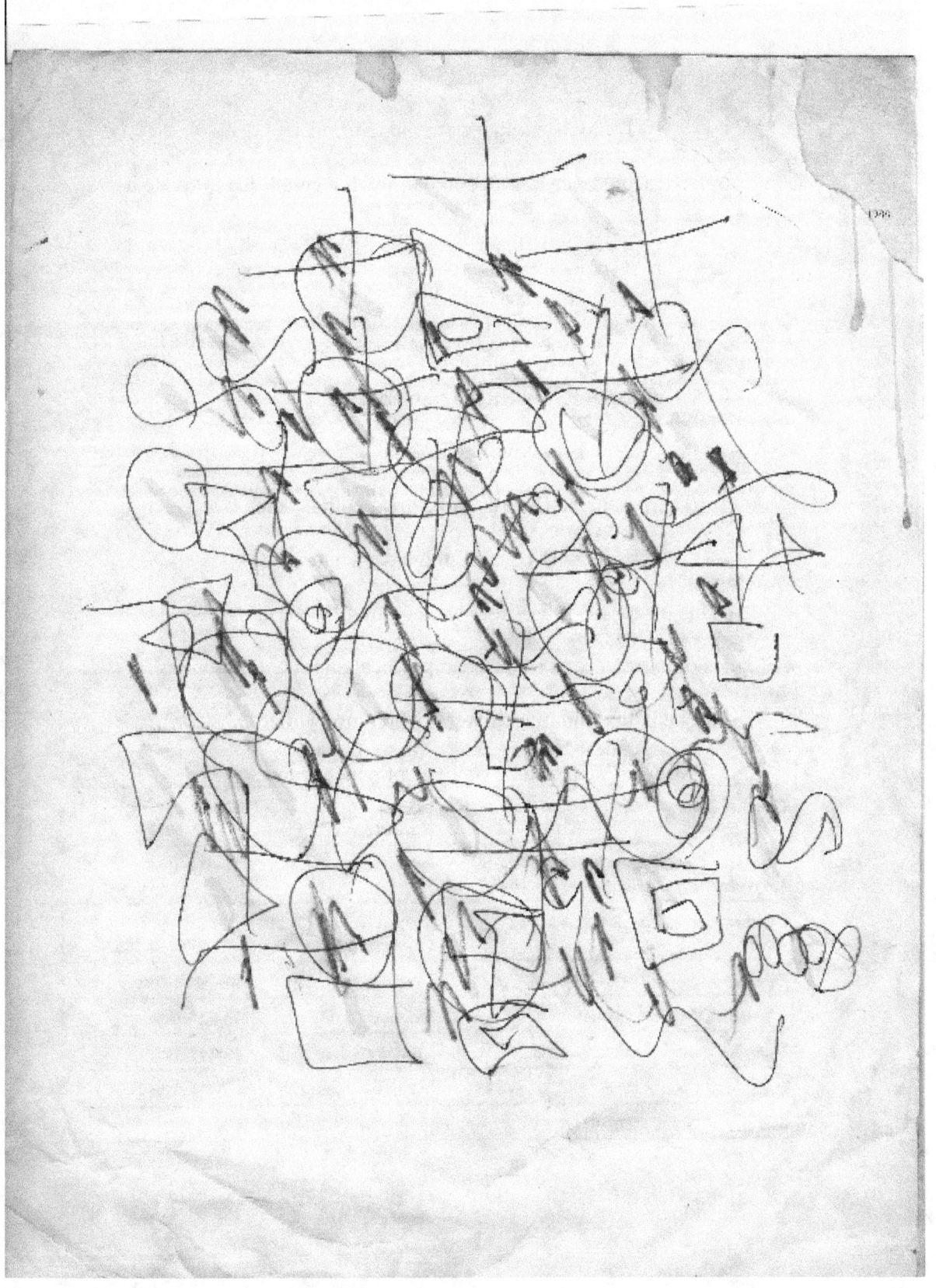

Today is Another Day

Sept 25

Today is another day of cognition

I seemed to have again once before come up with a great idea to battle it

I've been drawing dots on lines of paper

10-15 to a line

Almost twenty five lines

Every fifteen minutes

Today will be 2 ½ days

There in myself seems to be great enthusiasm

Especially because three days ago

This place was full of real bad cognitive symptoms

All kinds of extremely troubling bad physical and mental traumas

The house and myself were overcome by them

Now my idea of dots on lines of paper seems,

Almost 2 ½ days later,

To cause it to halt

'Sept 20

Today is another Day of
cogn. I seemed to have
again once before come
up with a great Idea
to battle it I've been
Drawing Dots on Lines
of Paper 10-15 to a Line
atmos almost twenty
Five Lines Every Fifteen
minutes today will Be $2\frac{1}{2}$
Days there in my self
Seems to Be great Enthusiasm
Especially Because three Days
ago this Place was Really
Full of Real Bad cogn
Symtoms all Kinds of
Extremly troubling Bad
physical ann mental
~~traumas~~ traumas the
House ann myself were
overcome By then Now
~~this~~ my Idea of Dots
on Lines of Paper seems
almost 2-3 $2\frac{1}{2}$ Days Later
to cause it to Halt

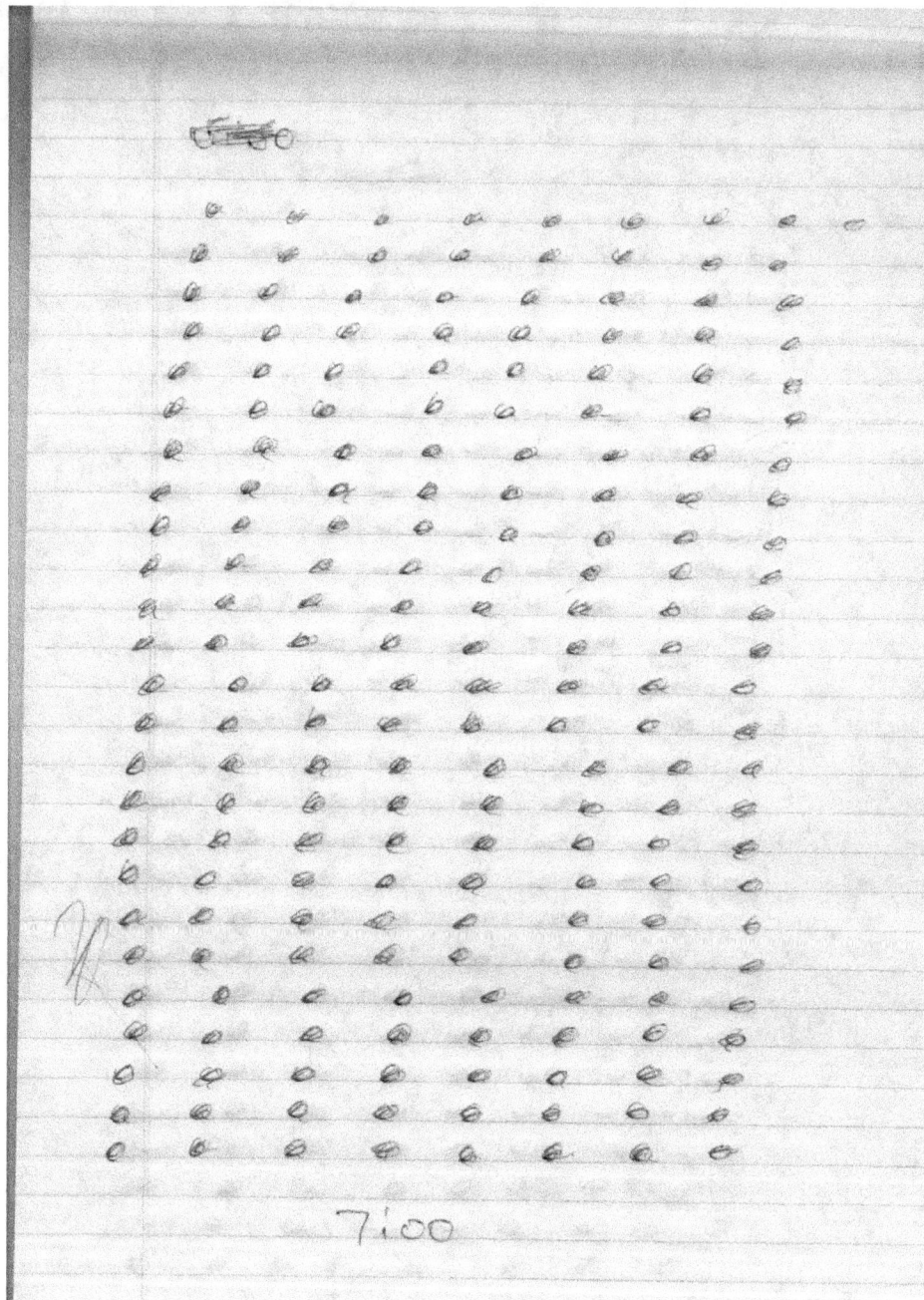

7:00

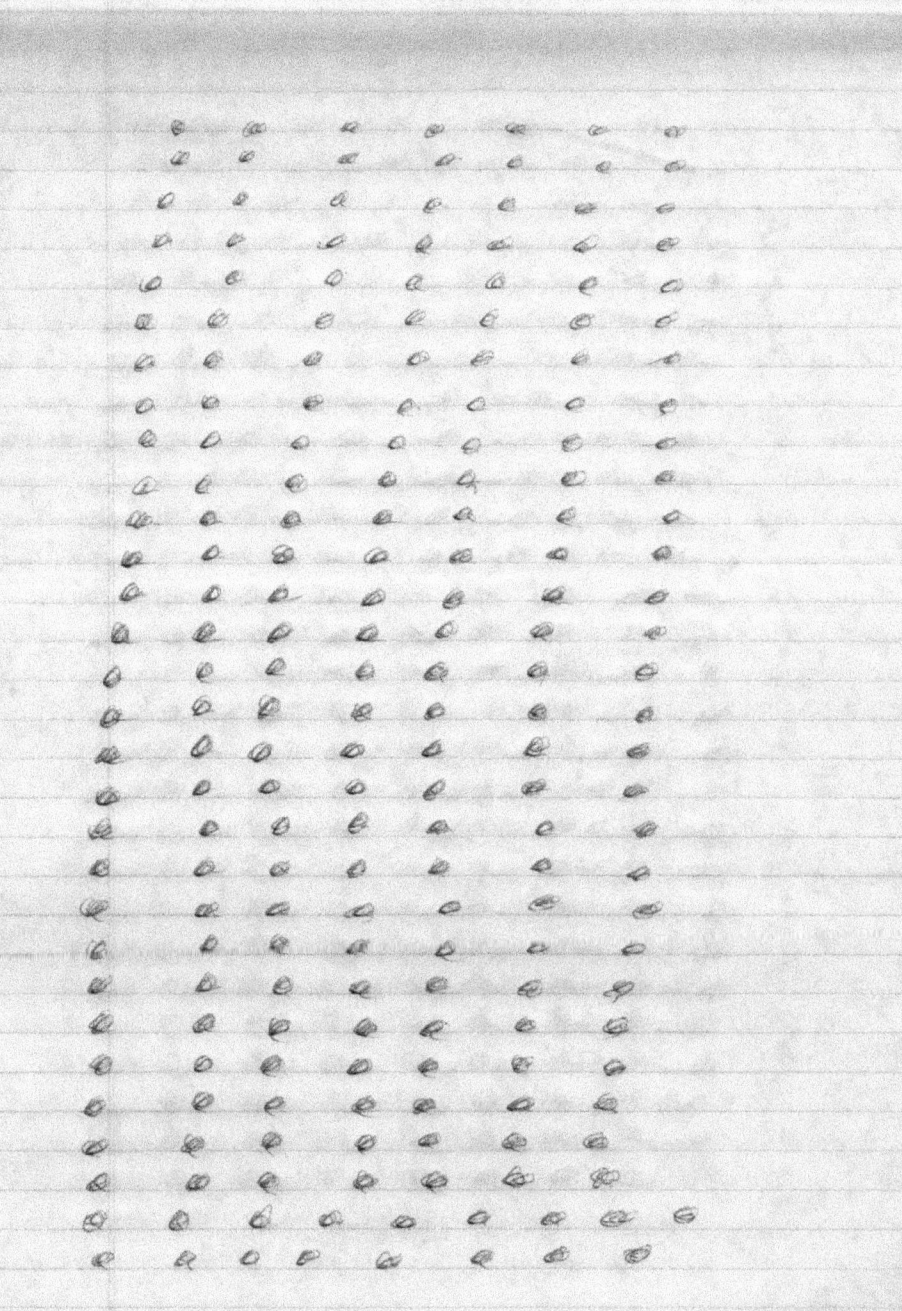

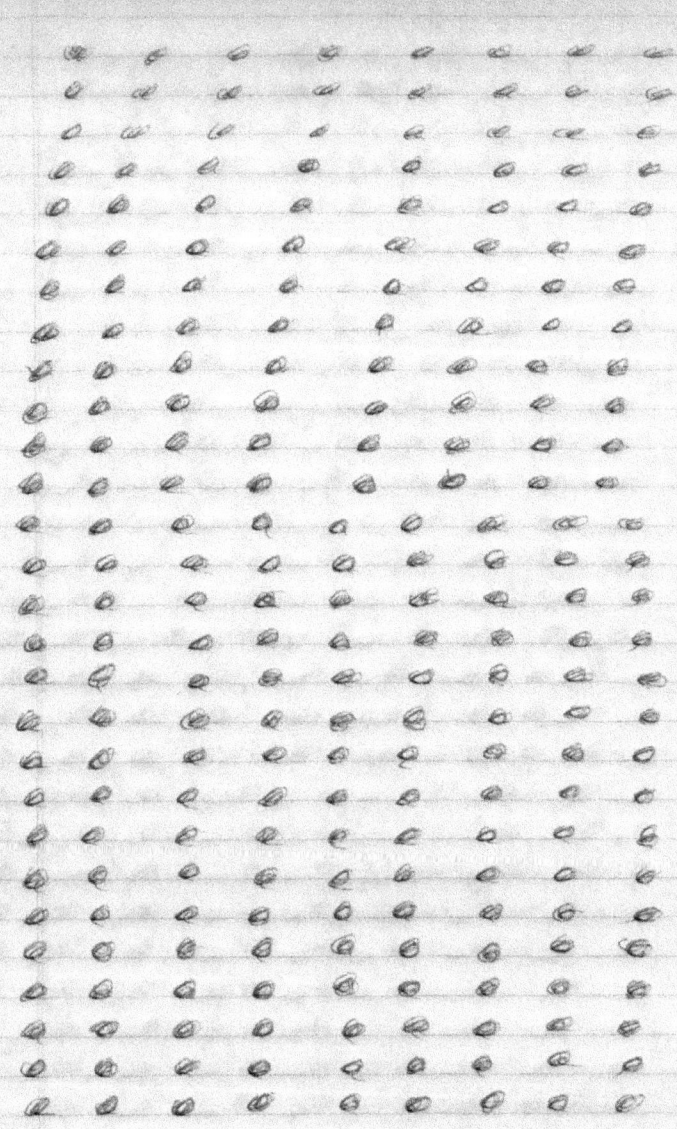

7:45

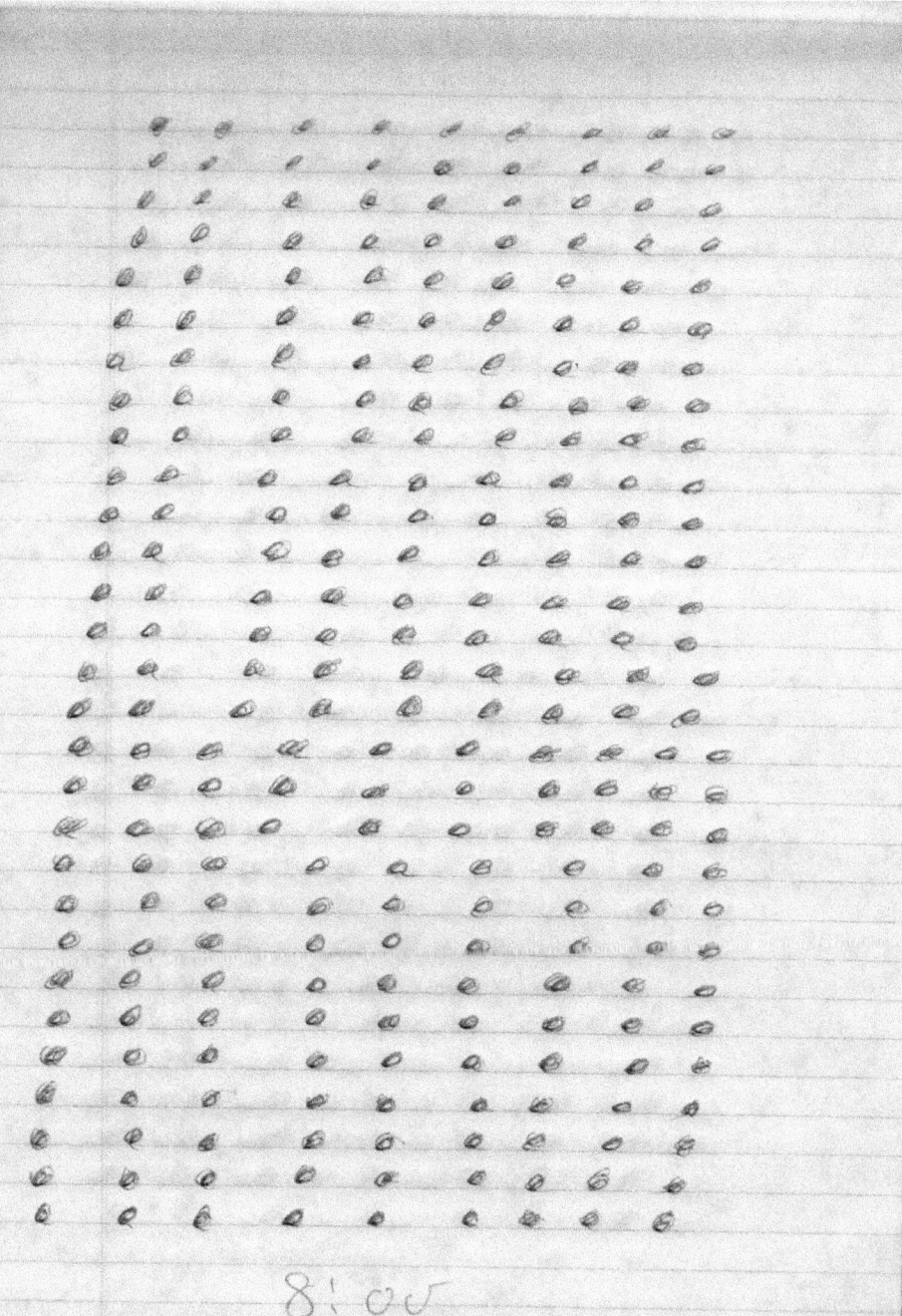

8:05

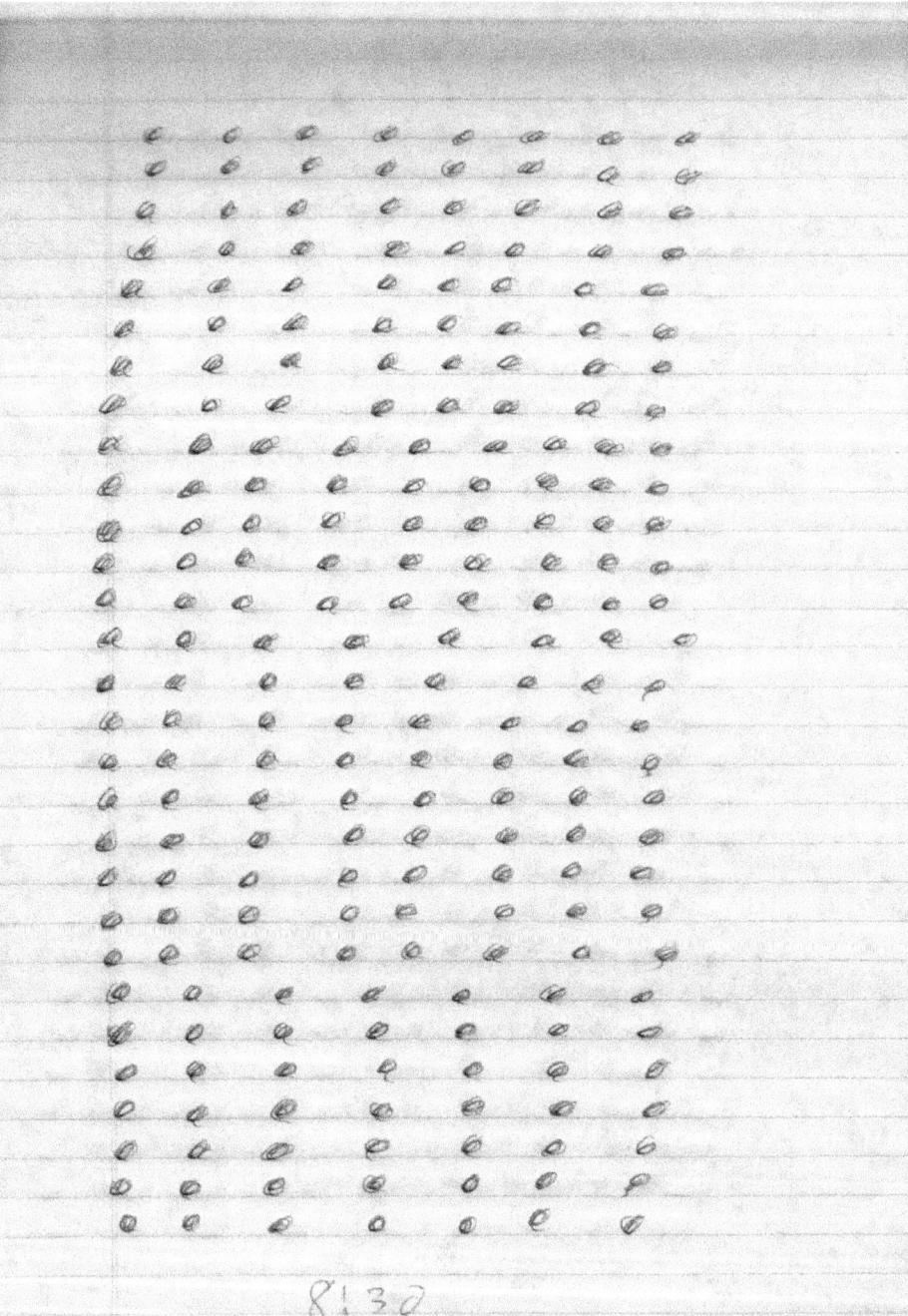

8:30

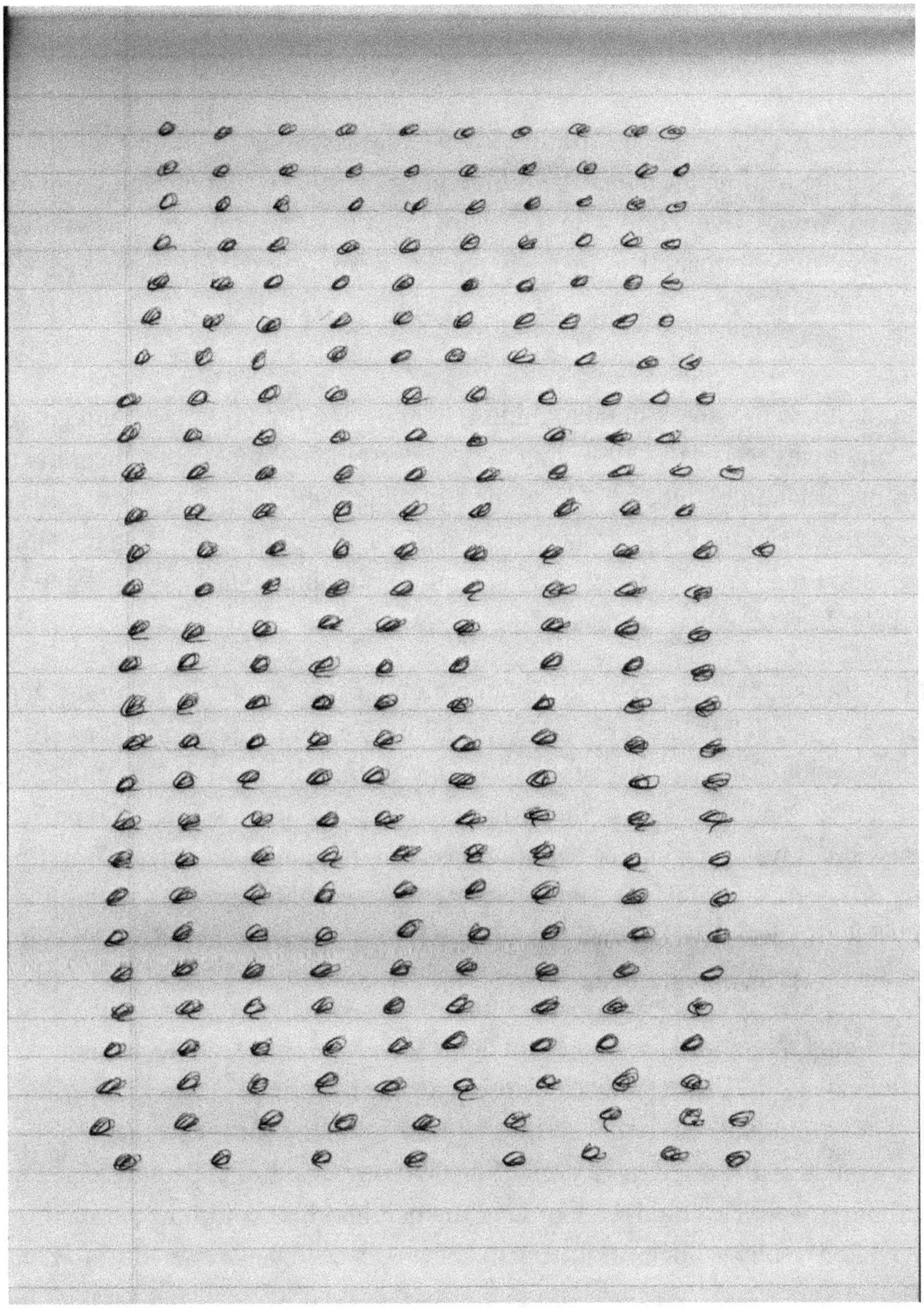

Trying to Save Fred

My parents were at a point where they didn't know what else they could do for Fred. He needed to somehow find the help on his own. The problem is that most schizophrenics don't think that there is anything wrong. They simply do not believe that they are sick. Fred was still in the apartment, and we moved to another area. My parents went to see Fred a few times a week. If he wasn't home, they would drive around and look for him or wait in the parking lot for him to return.

This went on for a few months. But then, things changed and Fred finally would get the help he needed. One night we received a call from a very understanding nurse at the hospital explaining that Fred had been standing in the middle of the street just staring up at the sky. Because he was looked homeless and had the socks around his wrists, the police took him to a hospital and they admitted him, and Fred agreed to treatment. The nurse explained that this was a good thing because Fred would get the help he needed.

It turns out that the nurse was right. After about a month or so of intensive therapy and the right medications, Fred was a changed person. He was taking Prolixin injections every six weeks and it seems to be working. The only downfall was trying to find the right dosage and sometimes Fred would get dizzy and fall because the drug causes low blood pressure. The medication part was a bit scary, but it was amazing to see him transform into a neat and clean looking guy. He stayed up in north Jersey for a while, and he was actually capable of taking the train down to visit us a few days a week. He became concerned with his treatment and would panic if he thought he would miss an appointment.

From that point on, I never saw Fred angry or aggressive again. In fact, he became very docile and gentle. He and my father became very close over the next few years and they became inseparable. They would talk for hours and were good company for each other. Soon after, Fred moved down with us and seemed to be doing fine. We now lived in the south Jersey area and Fred adjusted fairly well. He could walk around the neighborhood or go to the store or Wawa's for coffee. He liked to buy scratch off lottery tickets and would walk everyday and buy one.

But even in Fred's best moments, the schizophrenia still showed. He was smoking and drinking coffee excessively and still very hyperactive. He often spoke loudly and if he was excited, the volume would rise. He still didn't care about his appearance, and he could he could still become agitated easily. I have often read of the schizophrenics that sometimes go on to live a fairly normal life, including marriage, holding down a job and having children of their own. This was not an option for Fred, and for so many like him, the daily struggles of this illness never, ever go away. It is a constant fight and I'm sorry to say, in Fred's case, until the day he died, the schizophrenia was relentless.

Families caring for a loved one should keep this in mind. You have to accept that what you have may just be the best that you will ever have. We are truly grateful for the time that we had with Fred, especially the last few years. I think that we had reached a place of comfort with Fred, and he knew that he was safe with us. That is one of the most important issues that we needed to show Fred-that he was safe. Routine is life for some schizophrenics, and Fred didn't handle change well.

Although his symptoms were always part of him, he had days that he managed to control them. You take what you can and accept it, as hard as that might be.

Every Morning

Entry Sept 20 thurs

II Every morning I get
up wake up in my Bed
worry about my legs going
Downstairs getting coffee
my cigerette and sittin
Down and having my
gag syndrome come on
shortly after I sit Down
which is the present
primary Bad thing of
my mornings than after
I sat Down had my coffee
and cigarette it comes on
suddenly and lasts the Day
morning is ruined in
20 seconds there are
other Primary Points
of Bad Reaction
my Bed seems like
it Being Frozen with me
in it which causes
it to Bec. Become
uncomfortable laying
Down which causes anger
~~strikethrough~~ and causes
many a Bad reaction
in me to Points of
frustration and the
Horrible Episodial ~~traumas~~
traumas of the Evening

Entry Sept 25

Every morning I get up, wake up in my bed

Worry about my legs going downstairs

Getting coffee, my cigarette and sitting down

And having my gag syndrome

Come on shortly after I sit down

Which is the present primary bad thing of my mornings

Then after I sat down and had my coffee and cigarette

It comes on suddenly and lasts the day

Morning is ruined in twenty seconds

There are other primary points of a bad reaction

My bed seems like it is being frozen with me in it

Which causes it to become uncomfortable laying down

Which causes anger

And causes many a bad reaction in me

To points of frustration

And the horrible episodic (?) traumas of the evening

11:06

Different Locations, Different Help

Over the years, one thing we noticed was that not all mental health centers are the same. When we lived in Gloucester County, south Jersey, it seemed as though they were too busy to actually take the time to give Fred the attention he needed. Again, I am not blaming anyone specifically. The system needs work and there should be more help for families. I would sometimes bring Fred for his shot and I would drop him off and wait because I wouldn't be able to find a parking spot. A few times, it would be over an hour. I didn't mind, I knew they were busy, but there were times that they just forgot him sitting there, and that got me mad. I would go in and see Fred just sitting there and I would go to the desk and ask what was going on and I'd be told, "Oh, sorry, we forgot."

The mental health clinic didn't involve us and they never discussed anything with us. In fact, if we had questions, they would tell us they couldn't talk with us because of confidentiality issues. Fred continued to be docile and seemed happy to be with us, so we didn't press it.

Some symptoms of the illness never left him, though. He still smoked excessively and drank coffee all day. He paced nonstop and sometimes his days and nights got mixed up. They decided to change his medication from Prolixin injections to Trileptal pills which Fred needed to take daily. I remember Fred passing out one night because the pills were so strong that they made him dizzy. He begged us not to call 911 and he slept it off and was fine the next day. We called the doctor and left a message about the Trileptal. The doctor took him off it and they tried Seroquel, which proved to be well tolerated by Fred and seemed to keep the voices quiet, when he took it.

If you do not recognize the symptoms of an illness and you do not even believe that you are ill, you do not feel the need for help or medication. As we know, schizophrenics do not see anything wrong with their lifestyle. With Fred, he would say, "I don't understand, if it doesn't bother me, why does it bother you?"

He was starting to come out of this illness when he lived in Gloucester County and showed an interest in getting a part time job. His counselor set him up at a Bradlee's and Fred would have to take a bus to work. The problem was that the bus stop was over a mile away and there was no direct route for him to get to work. He sometimes spent over two hours getting to a part time job. We gave Fred a ton of credit for the effort and we were very proud of him. That was a huge milestone for him and we could not have been happier. He wouldn't let us take him to work. He insisted on taking the bus because he felt that it was a responsibility of the job. The workers at Bradlee's treated Fred with care and dignity and it made us feel good about the whole experience. It really was a great place for him to work.

Unfortunately, the Bradlee's he was working at was closed down and that left Fred back home again. He was really disappointed and sad to see his job go, but he was still doing pretty well. He would spend time with my father and they would go walking or just sit and talk. They became even closer and their relationship was that of two good friends. Until my father passed away, that friendship remained strong.

I Stopped my Counting Matches

10:55
sept 25 thurs
I stopped my counting
matches and Lay on
the couch For almost
a month Neglocted all my
EFForts I should have
continued them while
I & wrote I stopped
my gag syndrome dame
on Full Blast I got thrown
For a whirl like
Living in the cold For to
Long with un ample coats
or things of clothes must
keep on

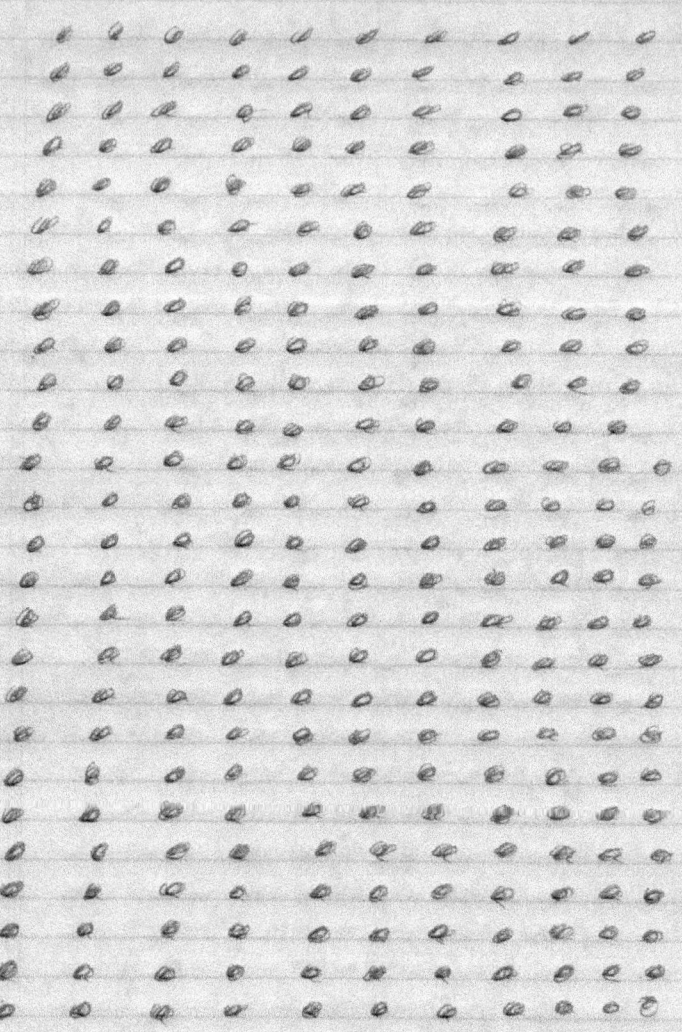

41.10

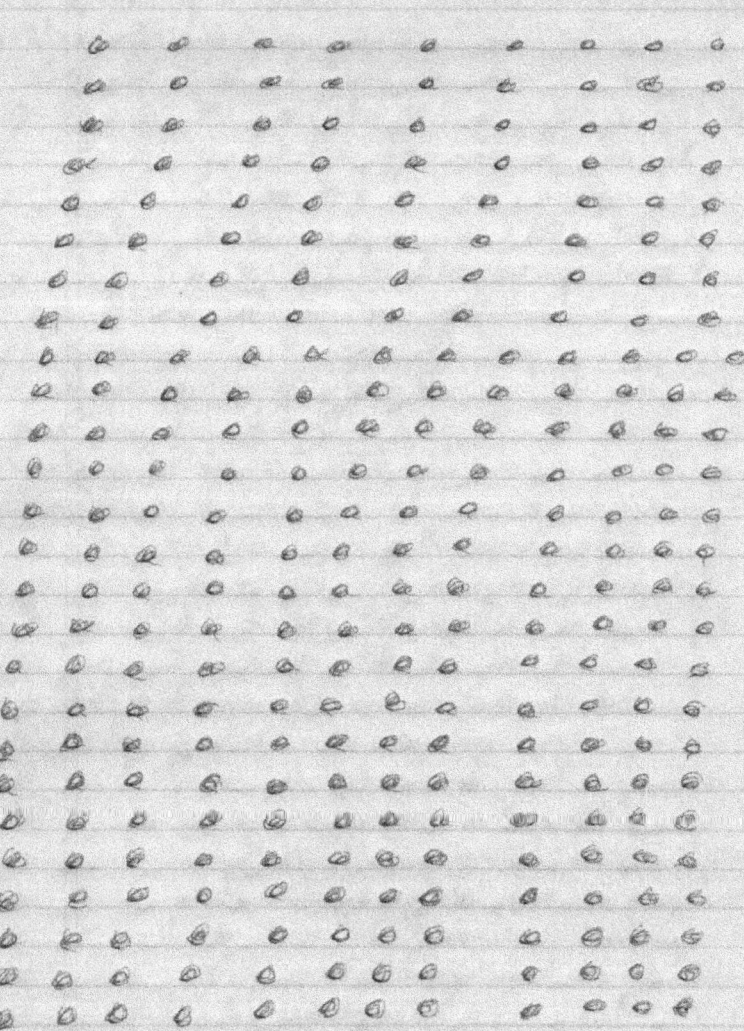

4:35

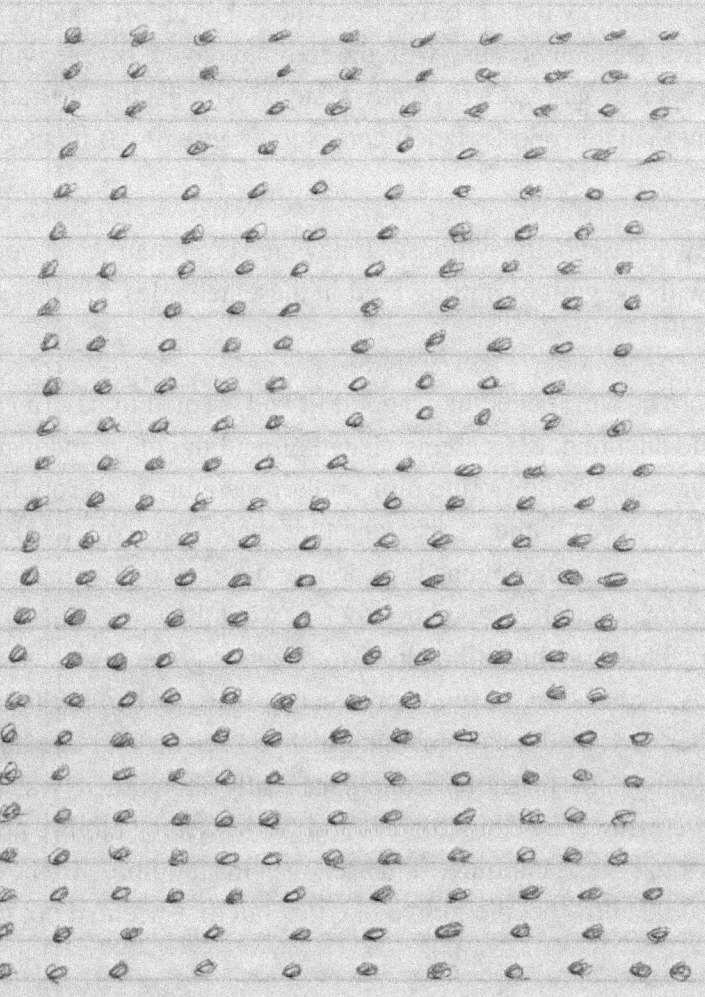

5:00

Halfway Houses of Hell

I am sure that good, clean halfway houses exist somewhere, but unfortunately, Fred was placed in a few that were not. It's a shame because with the right guidance, people with mental illness can learn to function in society again. As Fred proved to us with his job at Bradlee's, the mentally are no different than you and I when it comes to a sense of worth and wanting to function in society.

I can only hope and pray that the halfway houses today are better than what we had years ago. I saw my parents suffer with the guilt of putting Fred in these hellholes, but they really had no idea of what was going on.

One halfway house where he was looked like a good fit and seemed to have a caring staff. Fred never complained or said anything. My parents visited him all the time, and usually met outside. One night, they visited him and couldn't find him, so they went up to his room. The staff was busy at a meeting and didn't even bother to ask who they were. They went to Fred's room, which he shared with another guy. My father opened the door and turned on the light and my mother still tells us how she and my father just stood in shock at what they saw. The first thing they noticed were the huge roaches crawling all over. Two disgusting mattresses were thrown on the floor with filthy blankets. Clothes, trash, food containers, plates, and empty liquor bottles were strewn all over. My father described it as something that you see on TV, like homeless people living in abandoned buildings or a foreign prison. What really shook them was that my brother was lying on one of those mattresses. They ran out and got him some clothes and made him change. They left everything there, clothing, suitcase, even his toothbrush. They asked the staff how in the world they could allow people to live like that but they seemed not to care about Fred leaving.

Another time, my parents rented a loft from a woman that routinely rented to the mentally ill. My parents said it was a nice place and Fred had a small kitchen area and plenty of room. It was clean and had a separate entrance. My parents were happy that they were able to find a decent place for Fred after the horror of that halfway house. They bought him some furniture and helped move him in.

When my parents would visit Fred, it was usually at night and they hadn't noticed anything wrong until one day when they visited during the day and Fred would be wrapped in blankets because it was so cold in his room. My father called the landlord and complained. She said she would turn the heat higher. After a few days, my parents figured out what was going on. The landlord worked all day and she turned the heat off until she came back from work. My parents confronted her with this and she denied it, but whenever they went during the day, the heat was off, Can you even imagine someone being that mean and insensitive to another human?

My father called the landlord and said they were taking Fred home. They packed his stuff and since they couldn't take everything at once, they just pulled the drawers out of the dresser and threw them in the car. During the move out, my father dropped his keys somewhere and had to call my other brother to bring him an extra set. My father asked the landlord to please look during the daylight and call him if she found the keys. The next day, my father gets a call from her and she says that if he wants the keys back, he would have to bring the drawers of the dresser back and let her keep the furniture. My father was so disgusted, he said okay and arranged to meet her that night. They drove to the house and the woman wasn't even home. My father was so mad that he broke every drawer into toothpick sizes and left the pile on her doorstep. They never heard from her again.

Unfortunately, there are many more landlords that are even worse. Another problem is that even if the person has a great landlord, someone has to care for them. Unless the person has family to look in on them, they will most likely turn a clean living space into a room that might look like a slum area. Even in my house, had we not cleaned Fred's room and made him change his clothes, he wouldn't have bothered. It was still frustrating to find Fred's made bed bare down to the mattress in a matter of hours. Things that might bother you and I really don't matter to a schizophrenic.

As far as the halfway houses, I like to believe that much has changed, though I'm sure many like Fred's still exist. I'm sure there are many good ones, but if the area you live in has a hellhole for a halfway house, what are your choices? From a family's point of view, this is one of the biggest problems that we faced. If we wanted good care, my parents paid for it. Ever see the cost of these private facilities? There was a time when Fred was accepted at a wonderful place called Gould Farm in Monterey, Massachusetts. My parents insurance only covered a few dollars a day, so they kept him there as long as they could.

Gould Farm is a community setting and Fred said he had chores to do, that was some gardening and taking care of the animals. He not only enjoyed this setting, he thrived in it. My parents would visit Fred every weekend and they said he was doing great. Gould Farm specializes in the socialization of the mentally ill, and they have a complete medical staff to insure every guest is treated according to their illness. At the time, they were very limited in the number of guests that they could take, but Fred lucked out and got in.

Unfortunately, the cost was too high for my parents to handle and after maybe six months, they had to pull Fred out. Although they advised my parents against removing Fred, they had no choice. It was just too expensive. Today, the cost is $335 per day but worth every penny. I don't know many families that can afford the cost. Most mentally ill are on either Medicaid or Medicare. There might be a few lucky enough to afford private insurance, but that number must be very small.

But at least we learned that Fred was much better off being productive rather than letting him do nothing all day, so we tried to give him chores and jobs to do at home. It's just another sad fact about the mentally ill that too many people don't understand-the cost of the care is something many families can't handle. It's not unlike health insurance, the more money you have, then sadly, the better the care is probably available. That in itself is shameful and this has to change or someday healthcare will only be for the wealthy.

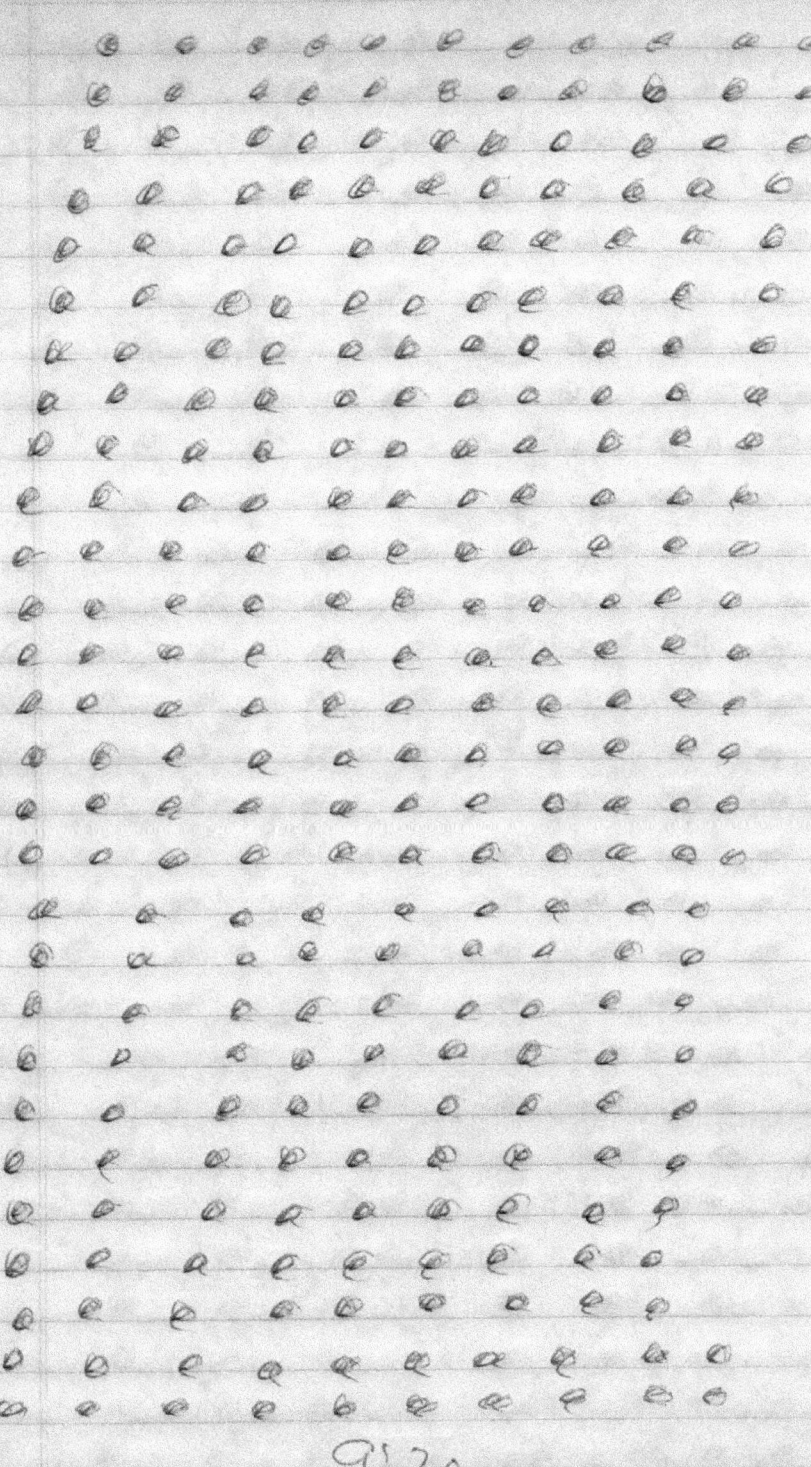

9:20

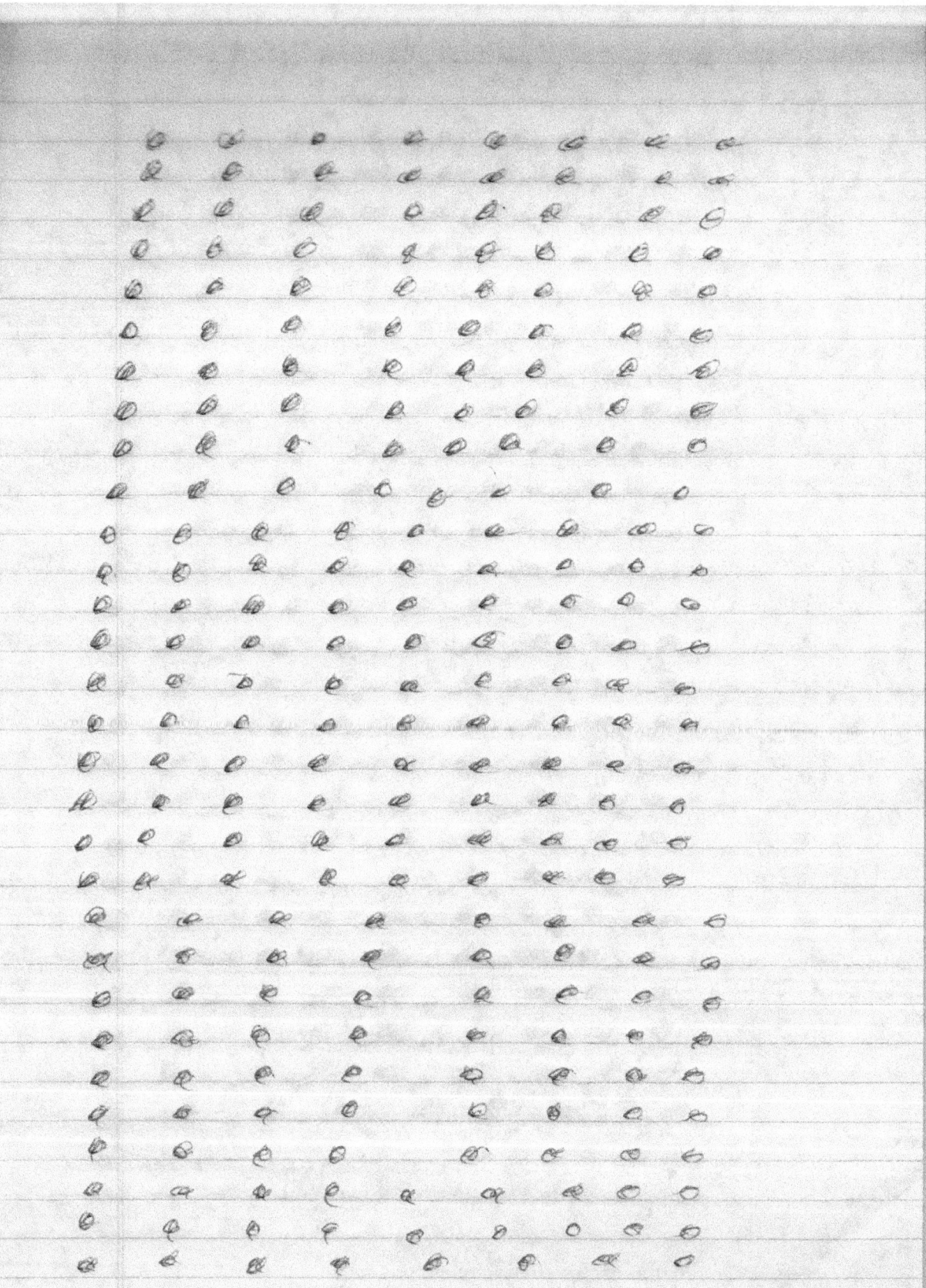

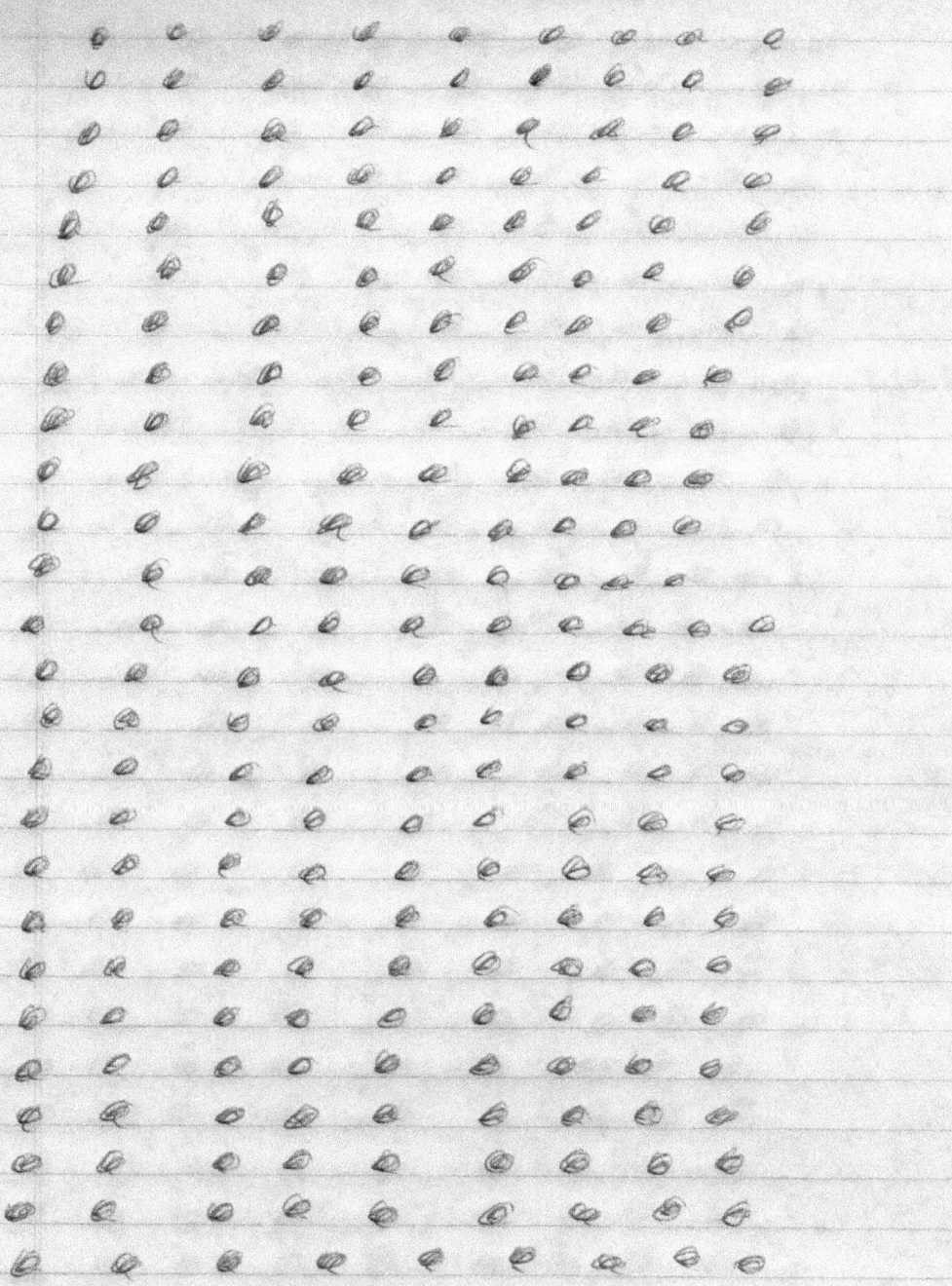

10:10

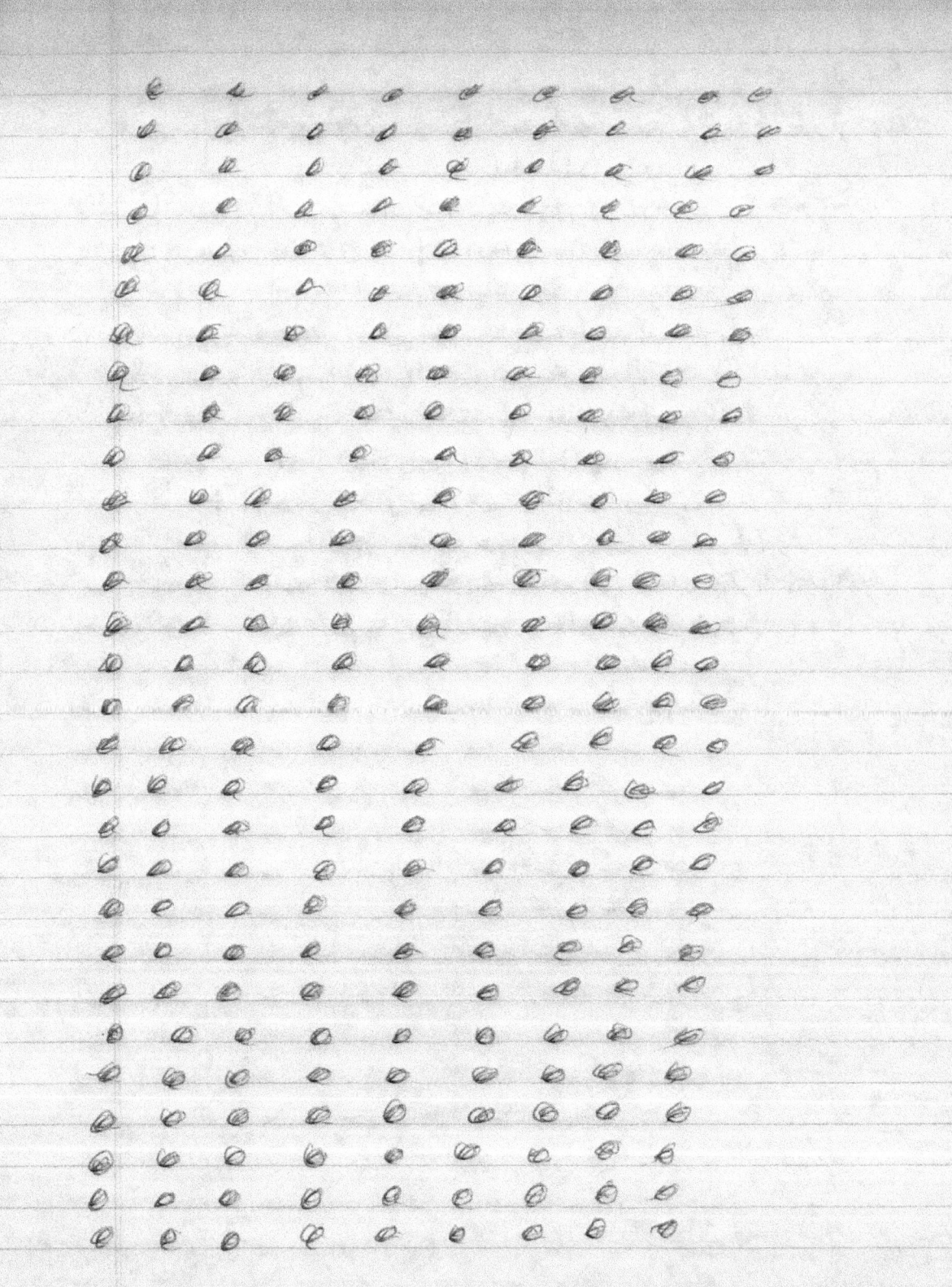

notes

No two days are the same

The one constant issue that we have always faced was that Fred was too ill to make it on his own and he was not ill enough to be in a hospital or institution. This is one of the biggest problems that a family faces. When Fred got to a point where he able to cope, he had to live with us, there was simply no other place for him. We couldn't bear the thought of looking for another halfway house.

As anyone dealing with this is well aware, a very frustrating symptom of schizophrenics is that they don't care about their surroundings, and even while living with us, it was a battle to keep his room clean and stay on top of his appearance and hygiene. We would make his bed in the morning and an hour later, he would manage to strip the sheets and pillow cases. He slept in his clothes every night, and we could never do anything to change that. He wouldn't even take his shoes off. I always felt badly seeing him sleeping on that bare mattress as if he was in a prison cell. Again, this is a part of schizophrenia that can't be changed.

Our hardest job was trying to figure out how Fred would process information. We didn't want to agitate him and get him hyper. If he was upset, he would pace all night. So we just made "suggestions" to him when we wanted him to do something. We might say, "Hey Fred, I'm doing wash and I need a few more things, why don't you go change and I'll wash your clothes for you." Or I might say that I was going to go mow the lawn and then he'd come out and do it. Depending upon the task, you might just ask him to do something. Most times he would agree, but other times he would say he didn't feel like it or he would say maybe later. When it came to making his bed or cleaning his room, it usually didn't get done unless we did the cleaning. Sheets, change of clothing, cleanliness and even comfort meant nothing to Fred. It's so hard for many of us to even grasp that idea, but it is the way of a schizophrenic.

Another factor was his intelligence. His IQ was tested somewhere along the way and it was high. Fred had a thirst for knowledge and he would often read a dictionary or encyclopedia. He would then repeat everything back to us. It was as though he absorbed everything he read or heard. He seemed to have a love for art and gardening, so we bought him books on plants, museums, artists, gardens and anything else he was interested in. He would sometimes walk to the library and spend time there.

In the year 2000, my father passed away. Losing my father was hard on us all, but it took its toll on Fred. Although he would seem okay, we knew he wasn't. Fred had not only lost his best friend, he lost his link to the world and reality. We tried to get him to talk about it, but he pretty much shut down. A few months later, while cleaning his room, we discovered a full bottle of his medication. He had stopped taking it. I called a counselor at the clinic and he said if Fred was off the meds for that long and was not hearing voices, we shouldn't worry too much. Even though he had a point, we were a bit wary. But Fred continued to keep his appointments with his counselor and psychiatrist, so that helped. Eventually, after some behavioral changes, they decided to give him the injections again.

A few years later, 2003, our house lease was up and I decided to buy a house. Fred did not take this well and in fact he insisted that he would go get his own apartment. It was a terrible time for us. Fred was angry again and he was very agitated. I am sorry to admit that I was so frustrated with him that I lost my temper and fought with him telling him to do whatever he wanted. I had no idea of the fear and hopelessness that Fred was feeling over this move. I didn't want Fred to leave us, and I knew he couldn't make it on his own. He needed some form of human contact and he needed direction. Left to himself, he would probably never change his clothes again and he would be living in filth. Being alone was not the answer, it was his enemy.

Eventually, he did come with us but he would not help us move. He slowly adjusted to the move and became somewhat comfortable. I later learned that change of any kind was especially difficult for schizophrenics. After Fred passed away and I found what he wrote about moving, I realized how traumatic the whole thing must have been for him. Even though he was very happy in our home, I often wonder if it was just too much for him. As you will read below in his own words, the whole idea of moving stopped him in his tracks and filled him with fear.

The best thing about this move was the help that Fred received. This community mental health center was a place like no other that Fred had been to. We called to make arrangements and give them time to collect Fred's records. I remember the first time we brought Fred there. It was at night and Fred had an appointment with his new doctor. He was also due for his shot. As we sat, a woman came through the door and introduced herself as Fred's nurse that would be giving him the injections every other week. We were surprised that anyone would care enough to come back on her own time to give Fred a shot. So imagine our surprise when Fred and the doctor came out and he asked that my mother and I join them. We were in shock! Never before had anyone let us be a part of Fred's therapy and we knew then that Fred was in a good place. We knew in our hearts that Fred would be in good hands here. This was in 2003, and he never missed one appointment for his shot. If we had a problem or concern with Fred, we could just pick up the phone and call and someone would always call us back.

Over the years, Fred became friends with Karen, his nurse and spoke very highly of her. Her friendship meant so much to him. Outside of family, no one else had ever bothered to get to know Fred. He once told me that Karen had said that he could tell her anything or talk about anything with her. I remember how happy he was to have that relationship with her, and we always encouraged him to talk to her. If something was bugging him, we would call Karen and ask her to find out what it was. This wonderful place is called Healthcare Commons and is located in Carney's Point, NJ. I am so happy that Fred was able to find these wonderful people and it truly did matter with his treatment. When Fred was going to other mental health centers, it was difficult to get him to open up. Even if Karen was out, the staff always treated Fred with respect and dignity.

A big part of the family life is finding a mental health community that cares enough to get involved. It's so important to find some kind of support or you will you be eaten alive by the same illness that your loved one suffers from. This is so important and I can't stress this enough. You simply cannot face all this by yourself.

Friends and family are not equipped to handle this, and you might find that some may stop calling and others don't ask. You can't take it personally, even though it may be difficult not to. People that do not understand mental illness can't possibly even begin to comprehend what your life is like. I could sit here and write all day and night, and still I can't begin to put into words or thoughts the struggles and heartache that my family has been through. And if there is a mentally ill person in the family for a long length of time, people somehow believe that you should "just get over" it and move on. Yet, no one expects you to "just get over" a family member with cancer or sickness.

It is equally frustrating to hear well meaning people voice their opinions about mental illness. Unless you have dealt with this firsthand, you simply have no idea of what it's like. That was the purpose of this book, to open the eyes of everyone that thinks they understand.

Most people are afraid of the mentally ill, and that in itself perpetuates the myth of violence. I remember one doctor telling my parents to treat Fred the same as they treat my other brothers and me. In a way, that advice should be taken by us all. Those who knew Fred and treated him with respect always received respect back.

One Sunday at mass, there was a young man (maybe 18-20 years old) seated about 4-5 pews ahead of us and I immediately thought of Fred. He sat down by himself and put his arm on the pew in front of him and put his head down. He seemed kind of jittery and always moving. When he stood, he was almost rocking. That was Fred, never sat still except when he slept. What really made us feel badly is that when it came time to wish each other peace, no one offered to shake his hand.

The point is, people don't want or mean to be inconsiderate or offensive, they simply don't understand and so they mistakenly believe that ignoring the person is the best solution. Yet, if he had been in a wheelchair, no one would have thought twice about taking his hand.

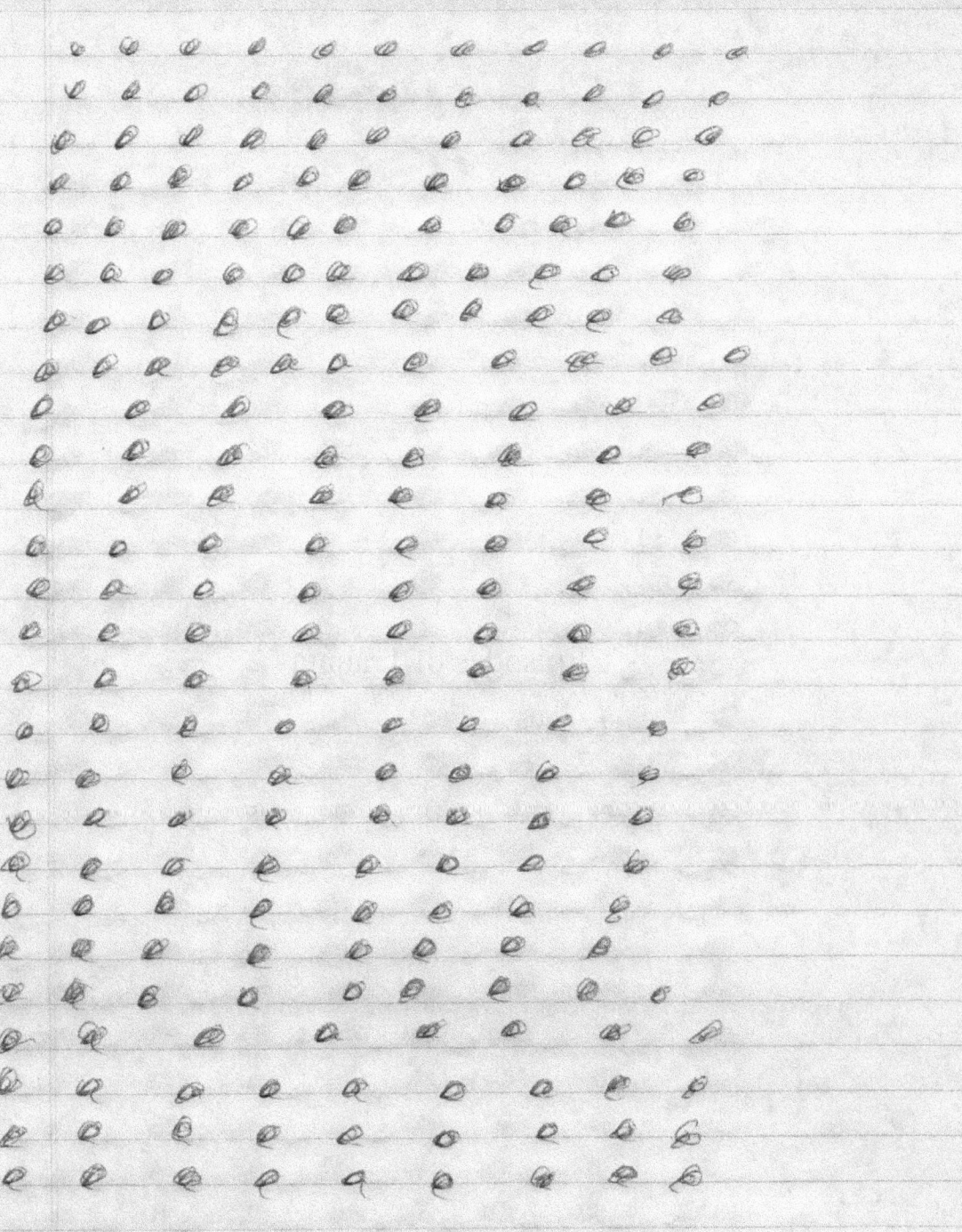

5150

Episodes of Trauma

Episodes of trauma
of cogn

This month The large
very strong and a ~~unhandle~~
~~what~~ unhandleable trauma
of moving was the topic
of cogn this month ~~it~~
It causes such a terrible
and hopeless Effect that
It sock a man or woman
to his or her Death
These Episodes are to
strong to handle so the
only way to Deal with
them is to try to cope
through it always thinkin
of the End Not the
Episode

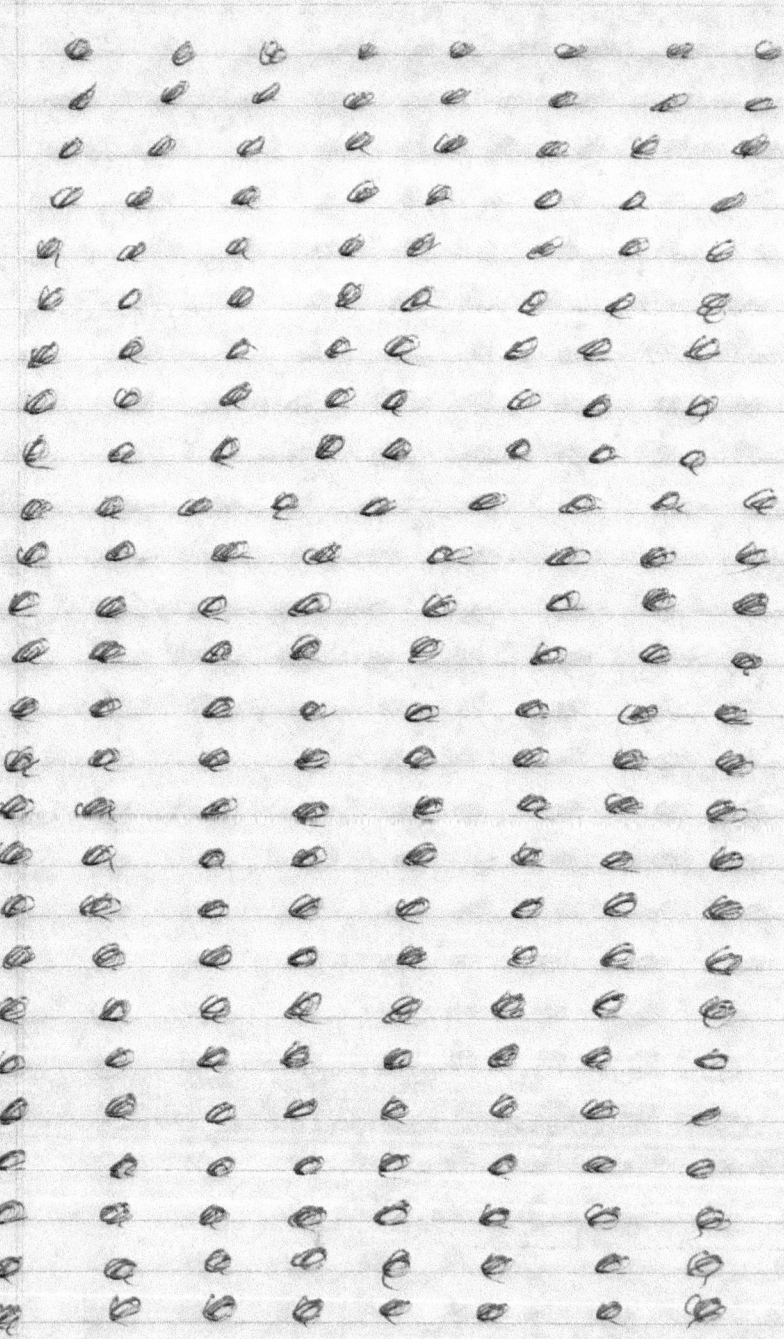

12:35

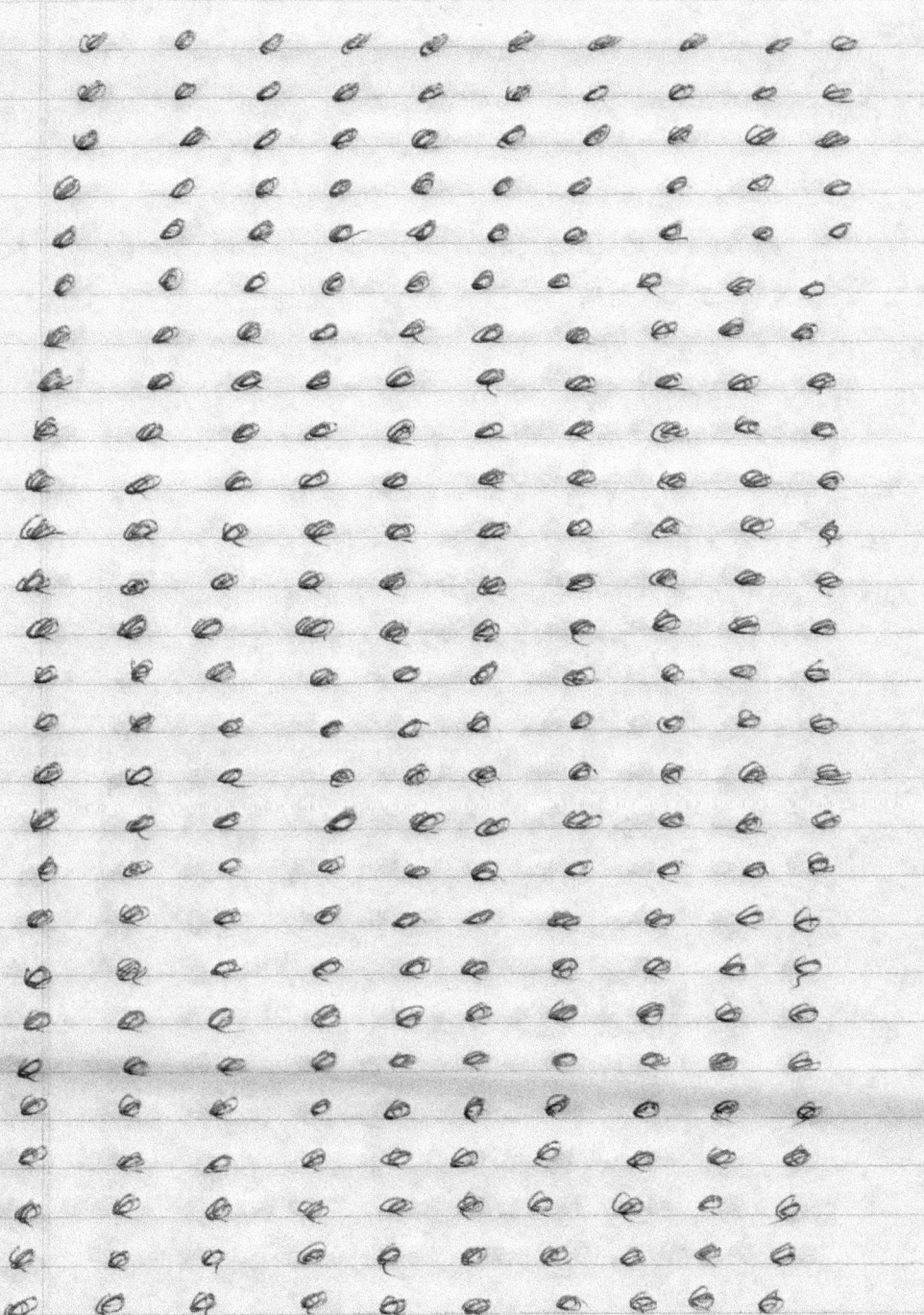

1:00

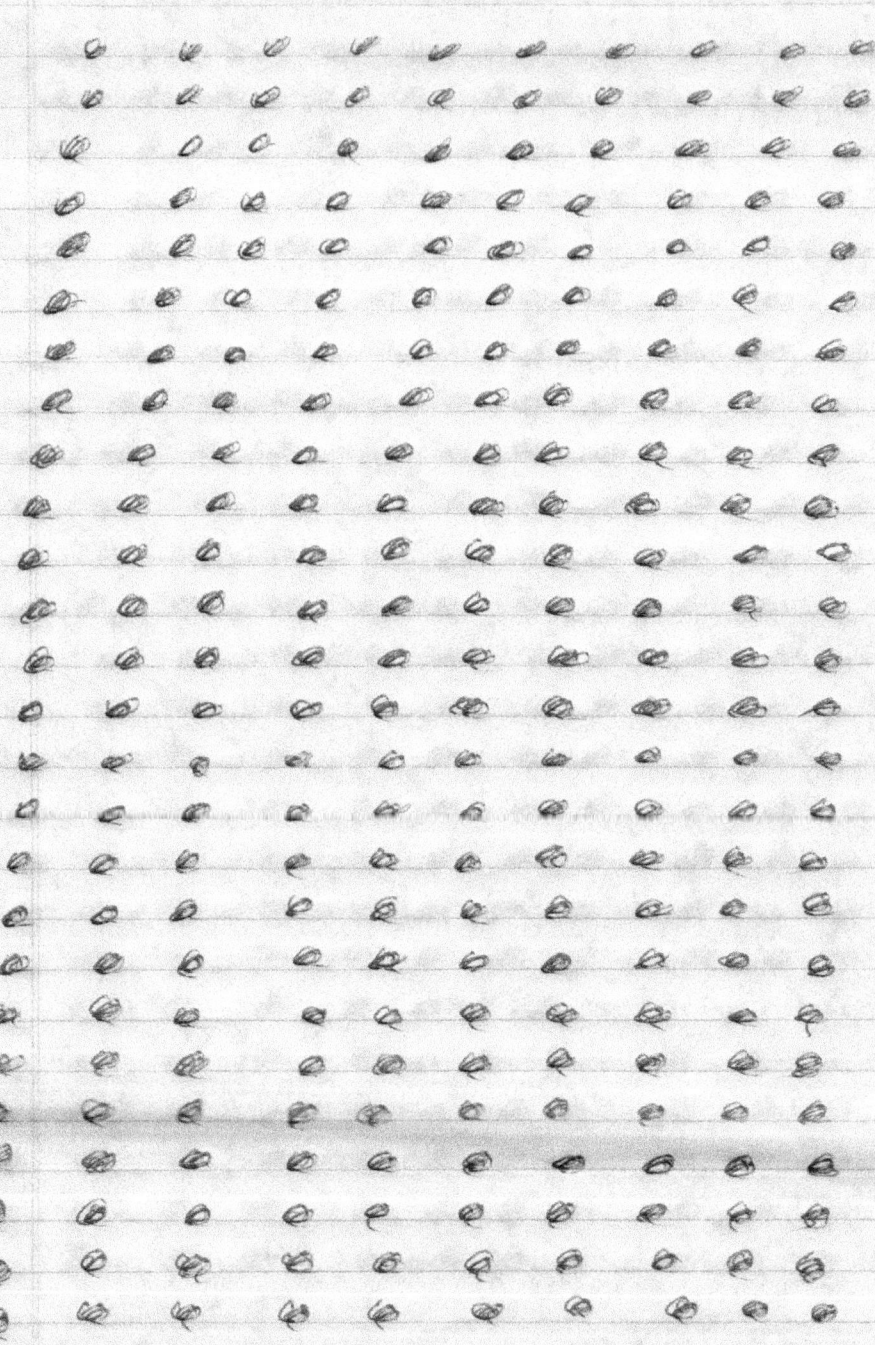

1:20

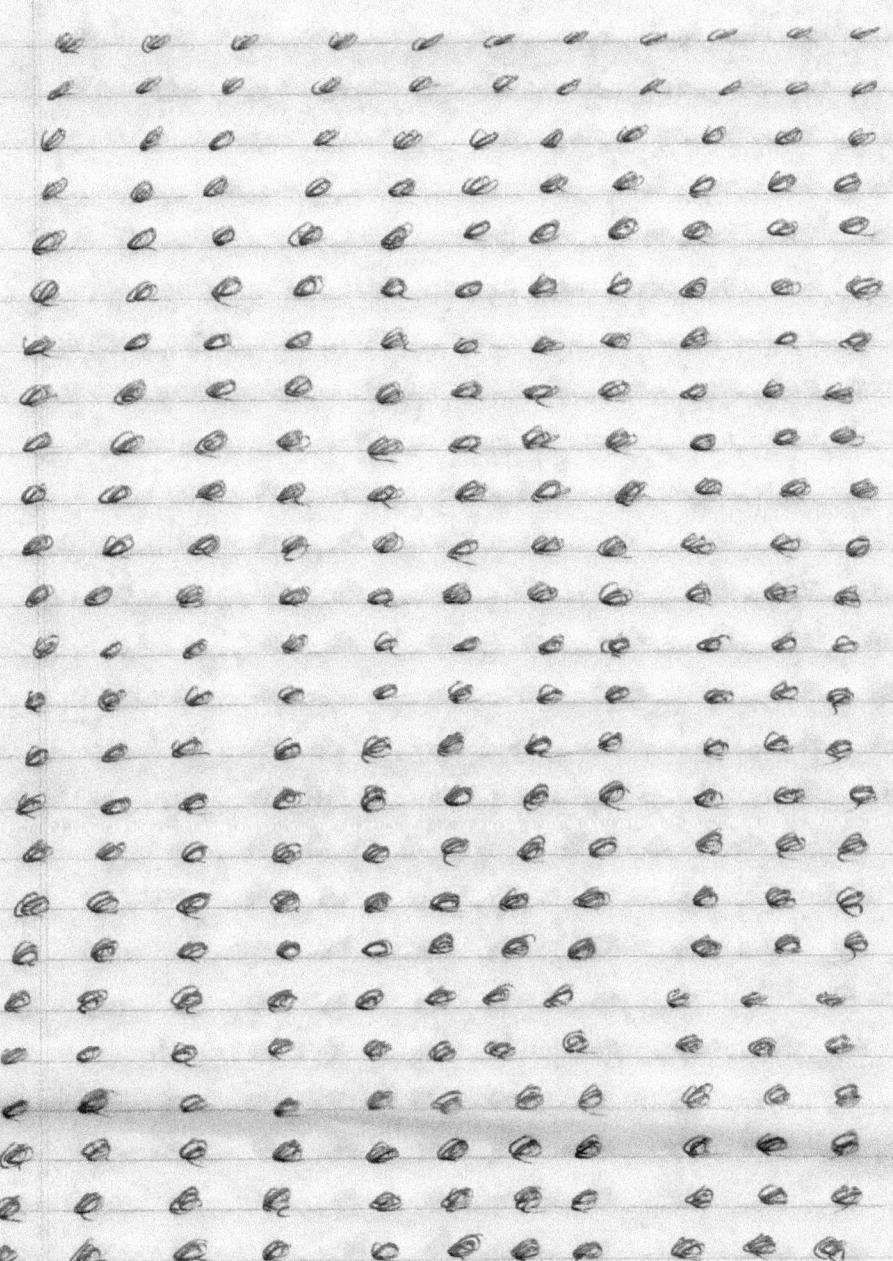

1145

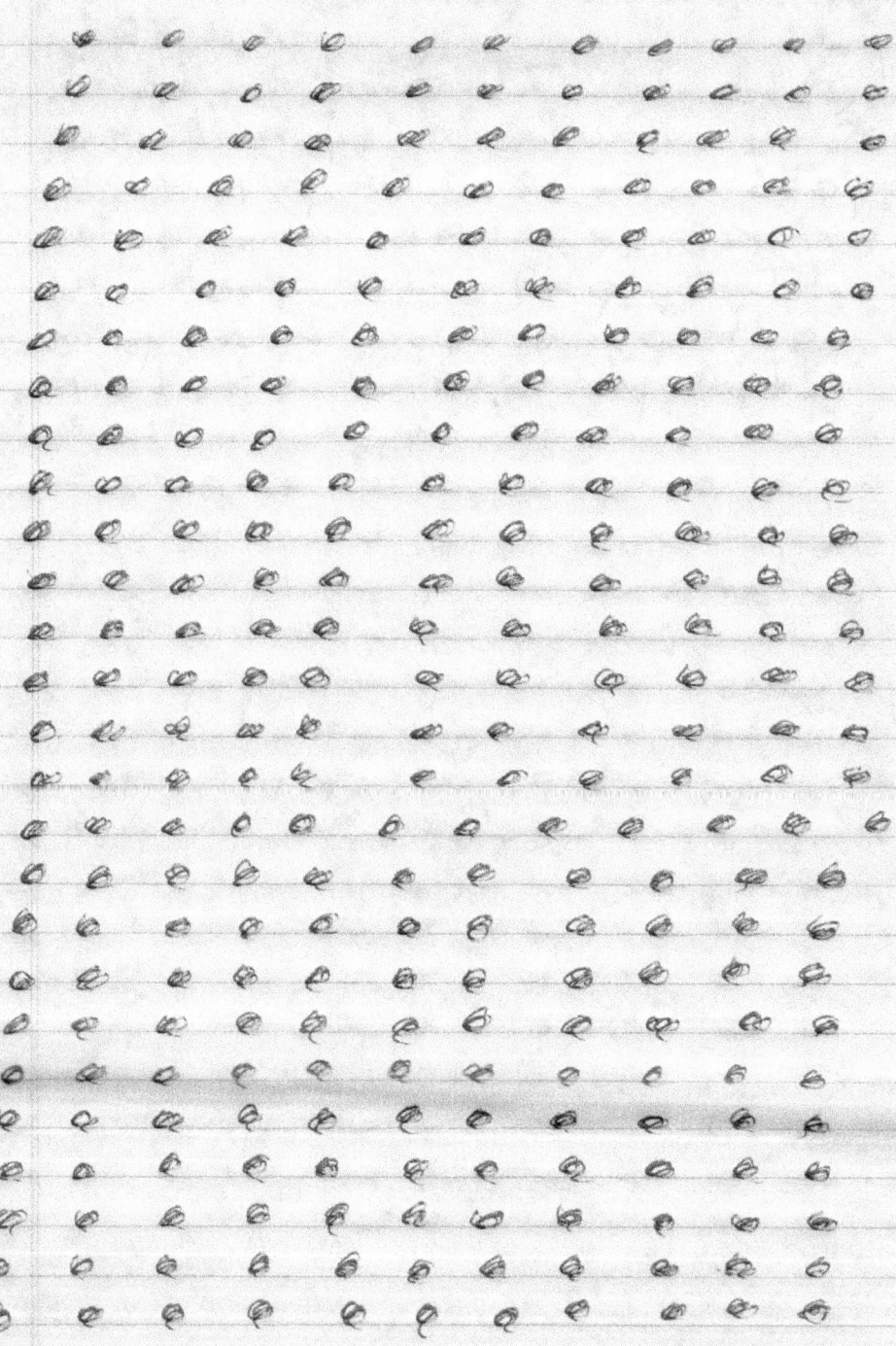

2:05

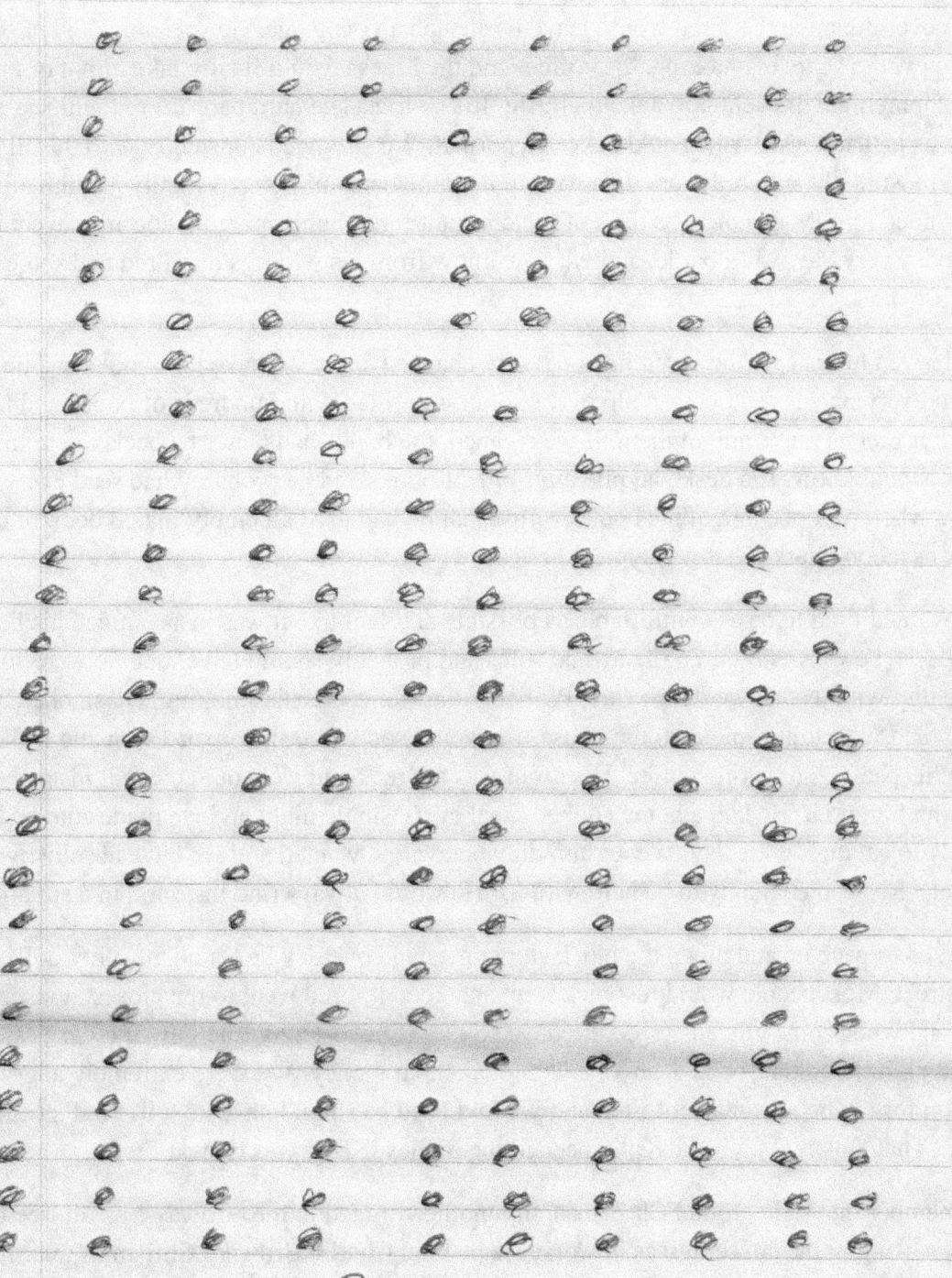

2i 3u

Tired of the Fight

We never dreamed that Fred would leave us at such a young age. He was only 57, but somehow we knew the years of smoking, the coffee, and the illness would finally take him. For many, schizophrenia will eventually take their life. It's so true. The hard part of Fred's illness and living with us is that we knew he could never be normal. We struggled constantly with this illness and Fred most likely suffered more than we can imagine on some days. It finally ate him alive and consumed him. Maybe he was tired of the constant fight. Schizophrenia doesn't have a remission period. Every day was a battle, and we now know from his writings that Fred had some really horrific days.

Fred loved to read and he loved books. Every chance we got we gave him books and he just loved every one as if they were alive. His room was filled with hundreds of books and he wouldn't let us move any of them. If we cleaned, the books had better be back where they were or he would know. His desk had pile after pile of books and he probably had read every one. We smile when we open one of his books to find that he had used an empty match book or cigarette pack as a bookmark. That was typical Fred.

We wanted Fred to be as comfortable as possible and feel like it was just as much his home as ours. Maybe we went too far, he had no rules and probably should have, but we were so happy to have him with us that we didn't care. Probably the worst was his smoking. He smoked 3-4 packs a day and we let him smoke in the house. He would sometimes get up at 11pm and wake us up with his pacing or making coffee. His room was a wreck and we would clean it instead of making him do it. He had a home cooked meal every single night and we made sure he had plenty to eat during the day. We let him do whatever he wanted and we have absolutely no regrets. He seemed happy to be here with us. He would always find the good in a situation.

He used to pace up and down the block sometimes and one day he found a twenty dollar bill on the street. Most people would just pick it up and keep it. Fred went to the closest house, rang the bell and when some guy answered, Fred asked him if he lost $20. The guy of course said he did and took it. I couldn't believe anyone would take that money. We were extremely angry at this person for taking advantage of Fred and we told Fred he should have kept it. Fred's response was, "That's okay. Maybe he really needed the money." That was typical Fred.

I remember that right around Christmas, my mother wanted to throw away a small tree that we had growing in the house. It was in worse shape than Charlie Brown's Christmas tree. It was about three feet high and the branches were half dead. We were kind of shocked when Fred asked if he could have it for his room. Of course my mother offered some of her healthier plants, but he wanted this one.

A few days later, we noticed that Fred had decorated the tree with Christmas ornaments and even put lights on it. Those little branches were bending with the weight of the ornaments, but every single one stayed put. I remember smiling and thinking how amazing it was that Fred always saw the good about everything. It wasn't a half dead plant, it was a festive Christmas tree. That was Fred and that was what made him so special.

Or the mornings that he would bring my mother coffee in bed and although he started out with a full cup, it was usually half full by the time it got to her. We just kept a towel on the floor by the steps to wipe the spills. We didn't have the heart to take this happiness away from him.

I know there are many people who will judge us and even believe that if he were your son or your brother you would have done things differently. One thing you learn about schizophrenics is that you can't change them and trying to might eventually make things worse. Fred took comfort in his routine, and we could do very little to change it.

Fred wasn't big on cleaning, but he helped us when he could by carrying things for my mother, feeding the dog and cats, mowing the lawn, raking and feeding the fish. Of course, it might take him a few hours to mow the lawn because he kept stopping for a rest and to smoke. Smoking was his outlet and although we would ask him to cut down, we knew that Fred could never quit.

We never once left him alone on Christmas Day, my mother refused to leave the house. On Thanksgiving, we would go to my older brother's but always cooked something for Fred before we left. Even though my brother and sister in law would send food back, we would still cook an entire Thanksgiving meal just for Fred on the following Sunday. I know we looked forward to these special times as much as Fred did. We hope that it gave him a sense of family values and showed the importance of our family being together.

I'll say it again, for anyone struggling with a loved one that has schizophrenia, take what you can and accept it.

More Dots and Thoughts

As you have noticed, I found many pages filled with dots drawn in grids and it seems as though Fred did this to pass the time. Or so I thought. Fred writes about his dot discovery and how it somehow involves the government and scientists.

The insight to Fred's mind that these drawings show is almost fascinating. The pages of dots are not identical, and I have to wonder if that was his plan. I arranged these pages in the order in which Fred had them.

I found Fred's descriptions of his illness to be shocking. I knew, of course that Fred suffered with these thoughts and voices, but I had idea as to the effect it had on him. This illness actually consumed him and pretty much ate him alive.

Fred writes of his fears stopping him dead in his tracks and that is exactly what his words did to me. It is unimaginable that my own mind would betray me in such a way.

It is my sincere hope that after reading Fred's writings that you might have a better understanding of what it means to suffer from this devastating illness.

What can you do? Well, for one, stop ignoring it. The mentally ill need our help because they simply do not believe that anything is wrong. If you have a family member or even a friend that is suffering, contact your local mental health community center and they will be happy to answer your questions.

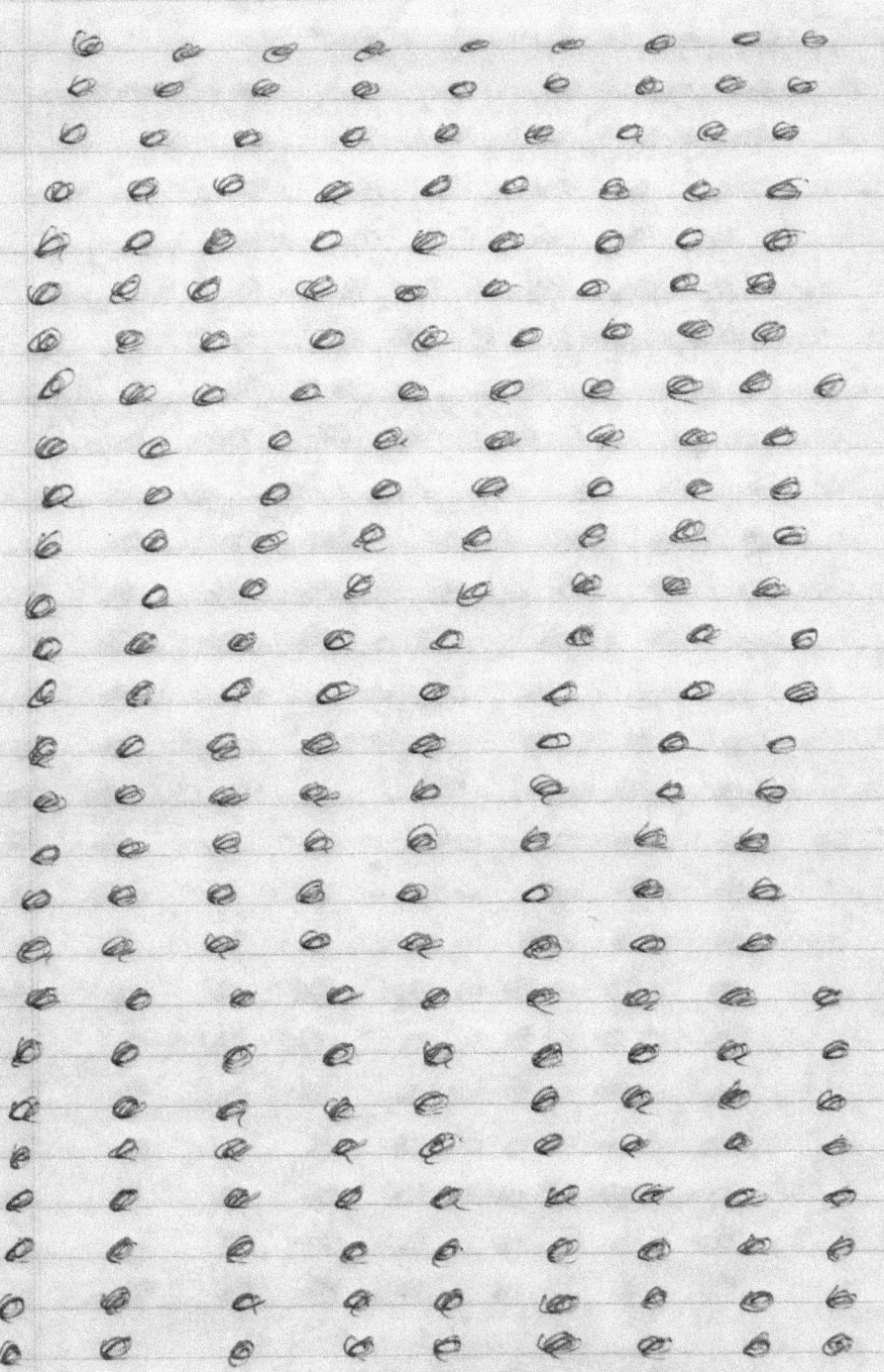

12:16

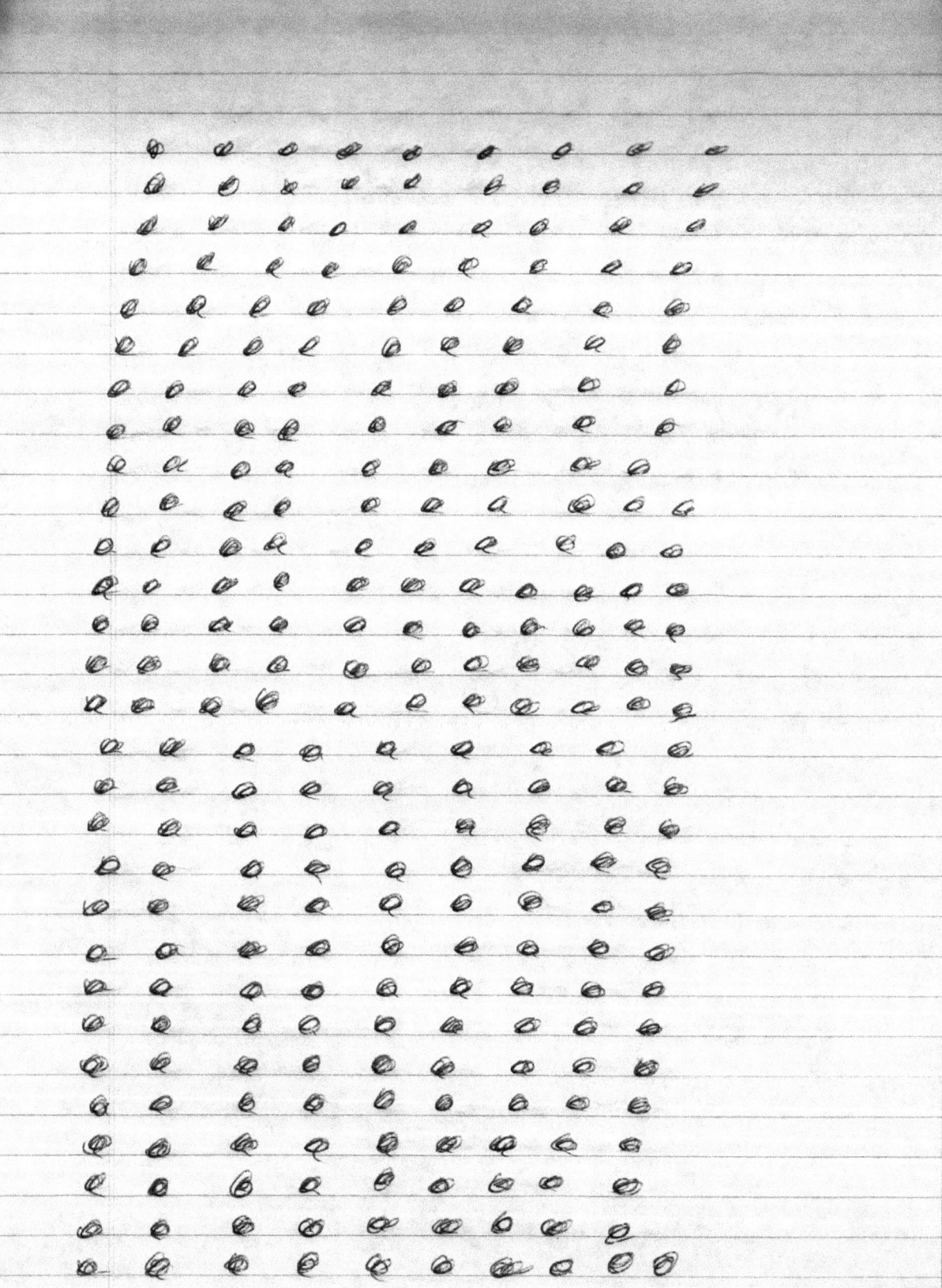

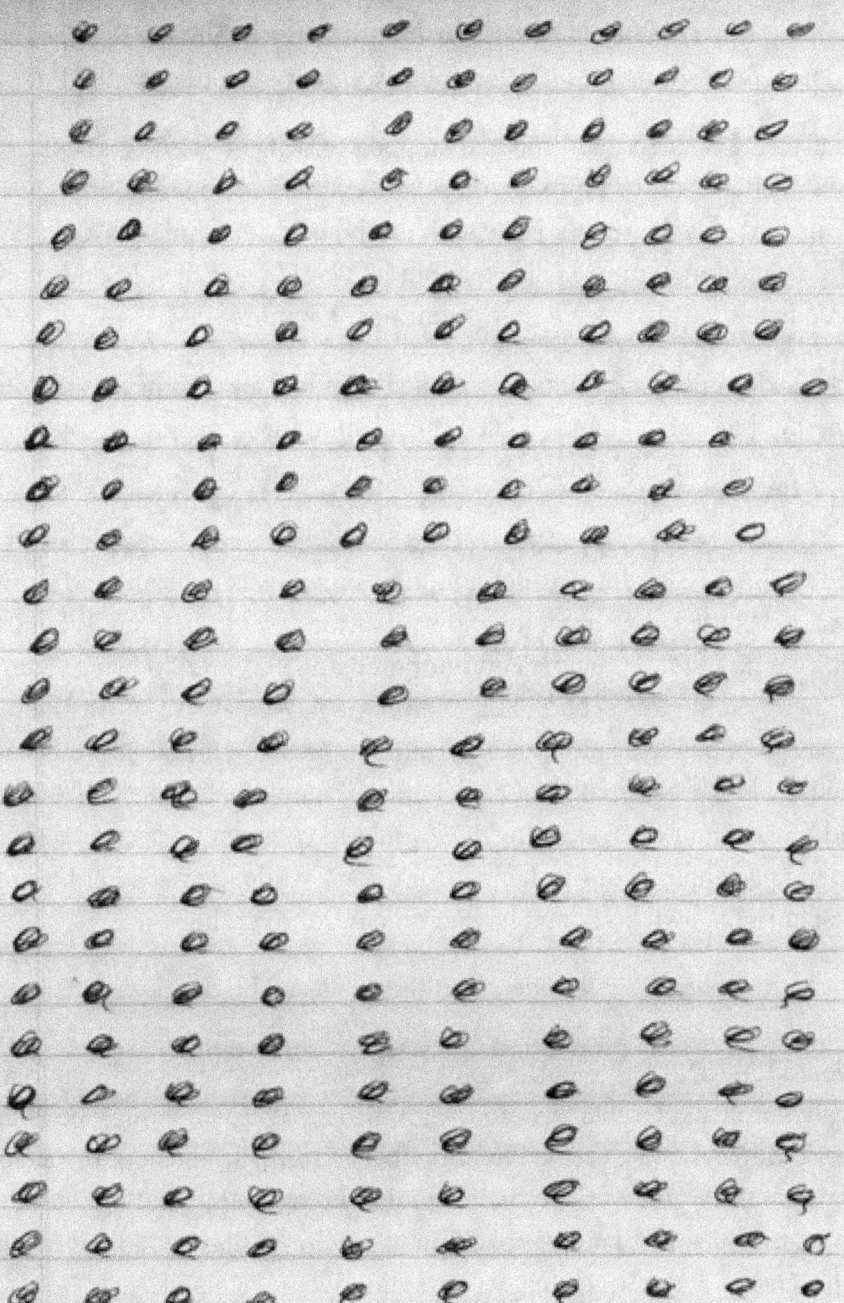

12:20

Our Last Days with Fred

As we look back, Fred's illness had changed him during this past year. His hygiene was slipping again. He went from showering every day to us having to keep on top of him. Many times, he would shower and put the same clothes back on. Again, this is the nature of the illness. His hair was getting wild and he would sometimes just cut it himself, but even that stopped.

While doing wash one day, I noticed that Fred had stopped wearing a belt and instead used a piece of rope. He said the belt didn't fit him anymore and even after I bought him new ones, he still used the rope. I knew it was the illness issue and not the belt. For some reason, he would not wear a belt again. We would buy him new sneakers but he would wear the old ones until they were falling apart. Foods that he always ate he wouldn't eat anymore.

On holidays, when we had family over, he would come down and sit with us all at the table for dinner. He stopped doing that last year and would instead sit at the kitchen table by himself. He just never seemed happy anymore and we had no idea of the torment that he must have been going through.

Physically, he looked terrible. His color was not good, his cough was constant and he was sometimes withdrawn. He started sleeping a lot and he was too tired to help us. Whenever we went food shopping, I would put the groceries on our porch and call Fred to bring them in. It was his chore and he was happy to do this. The Sunday before he passed away, he was helping us and after carrying a few bags stopped and said he was "Taking a break." Of course we became concerned, but he said his legs were bothering him. Unfortunately, that was a side effect of the Risperdal. He would be eating or even sleeping and would have to get up and pace. Sometimes he would go outside and pace up and down the backyard for a while. It was a hard thing to watch, he was a prisoner in his own body and he had no control over this.

Those who live with a schizophrenic will understand this. Those who don't will insist that they would have done something like make him go to a doctor. Well, it's not that easy. Whenever we suggested that, he would tell us, "I feel great! I don't know why you want me to go to a doctor. Maybe you should call Karen and tell her that you want me to go." Even though he is mentally ill, he is still a 57 year old man that can refuse treatment. The torment, the hell, the absolute terror he felt wasn't worth the arguments. We believed that Fred would wind up with the horror of one day having to go to a hospital, being hooked up to machines that would have to breathe for him. Fred made his choice and as much as we miss him, we understand.

On Thursday, January 10, 2013, Fred kept his appointment for his two week shot with Karen. Later that day, Karen and I spoke and she said that Fred had put off blood work since the summer and he needed to go by his next doctor's (psychiatrist) appointment. I told her that I would take him on Monday January 14. It seems funny now that Karen and I talked about Fred getting a flu shot and we laughed at the fact that Fred never got sick or even got colds. I honestly never remember him being sick.

He had an appointment with his psychiatrist on January 22. Fred had canceled two previous appointments already. He knew that he would be sent for a blood test and he must have been terrified.

Later, I found many prescriptions from his doctor for blood work that he never went for. It became clear that Fred was petrified of medical doctors and hospitals, especially during the last year. His blood pressure was a bit high and he panicked over that and it weighed heavily on him. The subject of going to a medical doctor was touchy, and we tried to play it down. We would say it was no big deal and that they would just give him a prescription, but that didn't do much. Once Fred got a hold of the idea of having to go to a doctor, he changed. He was so terrified that we didn't push it.

Looking back, I guess I knew something was off that Friday morning when I saw him. He looked terrible and insisted that he felt great. I didn't make a big deal out of the blood test, I just said if he felt like going Monday morning we would. I'm sorry now that I ever mentioned it. He must have been so scared and he couldn't process that fear or even tell us about it. That would be my last conversation with Fred.

He had been sleeping a lot and my mother had just told me that she was worried about this. Friday was no different, and he slept most of the day. Just so happens that Friday night he had his absolute favorite dinner, chicken parmigiana and pasta. Fred had a healthy appetite and could consume a double Whopper in under a minute. He ate like a football player and never gained a pound. But that Friday night, my mother said she knew something was wrong because it took Fred a very long time to eat. It was as if he was forcing himself. He was also sweating heavily, and it was January. After he finished and was going upstairs, he stopped and "Thanks Mom, that was really good."

My mother went to bed her usual time, about 9pm and as she went by Fred's room, she said that he was asleep. Sometime during the late night, he got up and sat at his desk, put his head on his arm and quietly and peacefully passed away surrounded by all his books that he loved so much. That's how we found him. He deserved that peace after a lifetime of torture. To die in a hospital was his biggest fear and I am thankful that it never came to that. He could never control his illness, but somehow he controlled his destiny. We know and believe that when he left this earth, he left all his sickness here and went to Heaven free from all his burdens and torture, and that is what gets me through the day.

It's very hard to look back and see all the things that we missed in Fred's behavior. We struggle with the questions and wonder why we didn't pay better attention. You keep second guessing yourself and wondering how you could have missed the signs. But then we sometimes feel that Fred is in a much better place, one where he isn't haunted by illness or sickness.

Mental illness is manageable for the lucky ones, but in Fred's case, it eventually took him. I wish I had more insight as to what Fred was going through mentally. I don't think that most people can wrap their heads around this. I know that I can't because I just can't imagine what it must be like to hear voices in my head 24 hours a day. It's a brutal sickness and hard life. So if we gave Fred some comfort, then it was all worth it.

To imagine Fred lying in a hospital hooked up to machines is a thought worse that the illness that he suffered. If you know someone with a mental illness, you know this to be true. They would choose to be free of the suffering than to prolong the misery by way of machines.

It's been almost 10 months since Fred passed and we miss him terribly, we know that he is at peace. He will live on in each of us in every act of kindness and compassion that we pass on.

We wanted to share the realities of a loved one that has a mental illness and to perhaps open the eyes of those that have never given any thoughts to it. Schizophrenia is a relentlessly brutal illness and it takes its toll on every person involved. But there is also hope where there is love, patience and tolerance. Is it an easy road? No, but for us, and for the great things that Fred taught us, it was worth the fight to keep him with us.

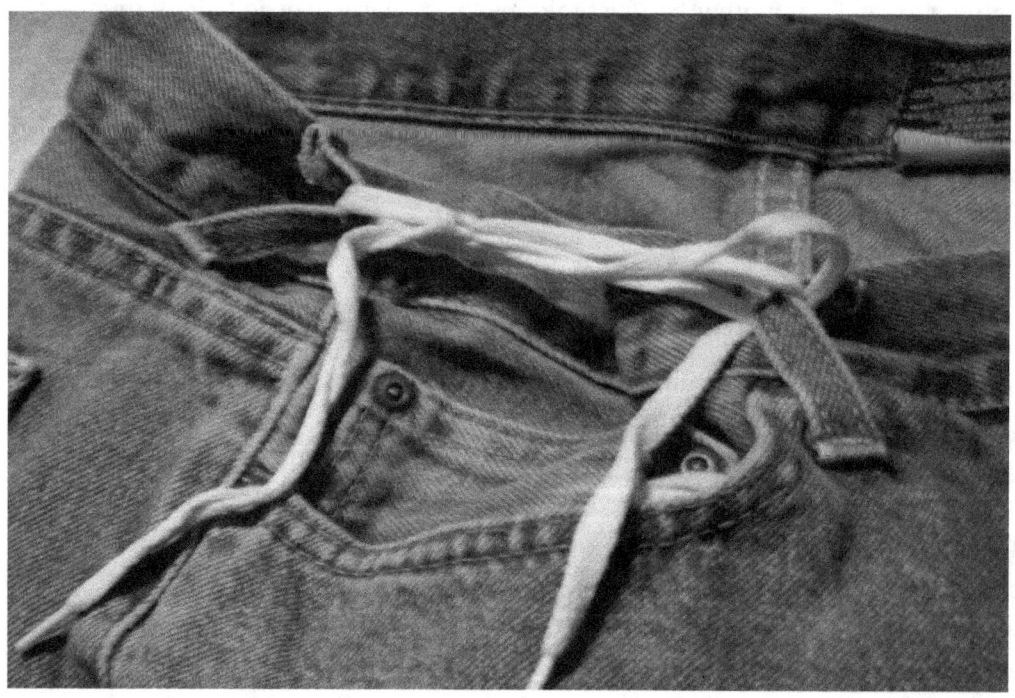

4/20

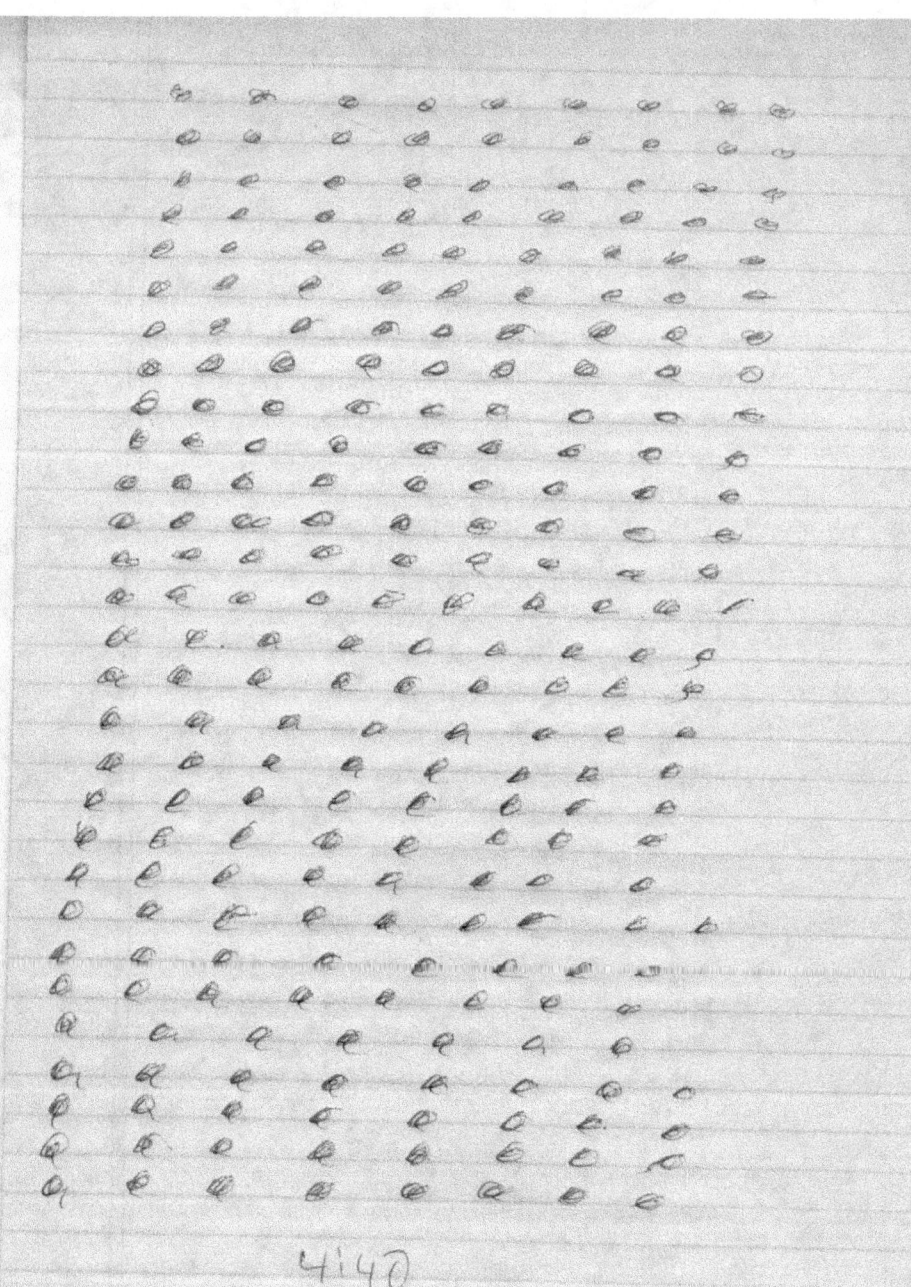

4:40

A Sad Goodbye

My decision to include Fred's original writings was an easy one. I wanted people to understand how the mind of a schizophrenic can be so complicated and so paranoid that it just consumes them. Many families cannot handle the day to day frustration and believe me, we had our moments when we wondered whether we were doing more harm than good. There was always fighting over his treatment, and we all had struggles accepting Fred.

One thing we know for sure is that there just isn't any place for people like Fred. Society is very hard on the mentally ill and many times they wind up homeless or living in filth. What's very difficult for them is getting treatment in a hospital and then being let out on the street because there is no place to put them. So what happens? They stop taking medication and the cycle begins all over.

When I read about the voices in Fred's writings, I understood why I found several walkman radios hidden within his drawers. It most likely had something to do with the voices that tortured him. By placing the walkmans under his clothing in the corners, he must have been trying to silence them. For Fred, voices were associated with radios and TV's. He rarely watched TV and although he did sometimes listen to music, those times were few and far between. If we left the TV on when we walked out of a room, he would turn it off. He didn't have a TV in his room, and he never wanted one. He preferred his books and magazines.

I know that there are professionals out there that would insist that schizophrenics can lead a productive life with the right medications, but I honestly don't believe that this was a choice for Fred. His illness was far too strong for him to handle. Doctors insist that schizophrenia is not a death sentence, and again, I would disagree in Fred's case. His excessive lifestyle was a direct result of the schizophrenia. But I do believe that everyone is different and there are degrees of every sickness out there. I also believe that no one should ever give up. In fact, I was always hopeful and optimistic until Fred passed away and I read his writings. It was only then that I truly understood how devastating and brutal schizophrenia really is.

There may be medications that quiet the voices in their heads, but there will never be a medication that will allow people like Fred to live a normal life. That's the brutal truth about schizophrenia. I mean no disrespect to the medical profession, but any doctor that believes a medication does exist that will "cure" this illness hasn't worked with patients as sick as Fred. That's the reality and the hardest part of trying to deal with this. As his caregiver, I could take him for his shots, cook for him, wash his clothes, make his bed or buy him all the books that he could read. But I could never help him through the torment that he lived with. I couldn't quiet the voices in his head and I couldn't make him believe that people didn't care if he walked in front of their homes. He had to deal with this mental torture every single day and many times, we didn't even know how bad things must have been.

Yet, we feel so lucky to have had Fred with us. It was obviously such a fight for him, and we are so happy that he fought for as long as he did.

Although our family is deeply saddened and will struggle will Fred's passing for a long time, we are grateful for the joy and goodness that he gave us so unselfishly. He showed us every day that even the most devastating of illnesses could allow someone to still appreciate the beauty of a rose or the magnificence of artwork.

Fred's passing has had an overwhelming impact on my family. We are now the ones that struggle through each day. We wonder if there was something that we should have done. Our home feels empty and our hearts still ache and will for a long time. We try to take comfort in the fact that he knew we loved him and he seemed happy here. We like to believe that in the end, he didn't suffer or feel any pain and for that we are grateful.

I found this poem that Fred had written, and it made me wonder when Fred wrote it and what he was thinking. It is almost as if he knew that this battle could never be won.

I thought it was appropriate to end this book with Fred's poem that he called "Days Lost." As much as I truly miss Fred, I feel that there is a new purpose in this life for me, and it involves sharing this story with as many people as possible. There has to be changes made to the system and more important, we need to educate people and change the stigma attached to being mentally ill.

Mys Lot

Occasionaly it rests
upon the soul
I have too paint
or fruit filled bowl
I found year prop
in my lifes pattern
but in the night
I flight my fear
in leaving my dear
Earth

Days Lost

Occasionally it rests

Upon the soul

I have no drink

Or fruit filled bowl

I found dear droop

In my life's patter

But in the night

I fright for fear

In leaving my dear earth

Getting Help

http://www.nimh.nih.gov/health/publications/schizophrenia/complete-index.shtml

http://www.schizophrenia.com/invol.html

http://psychcentral.com/lib/2006/helpful-hints-about-schizophrenia-for-family-members-and-others/

http://www.mentalhealth.gov/

http://www.mentalhealthamerica.net/go/information/get-info/schizophrenia/schizophrenia-what-you-need-to-know

http://www.helpstartshere.org/mind-and-spirit/schizophrenia/schizophrenia-resources.html

http://www.nami.org/Template.cfm?Section=Schizophrenia9&Template=/ContentManagement/ContentDisplay.cfm&ContentID=118290

Also, please feel free to email me let me know what is going on in your world.

This news story is a sad but realistic view of how schizophrenics are treated. Happens more than it should.

http://www.foxnews.com/politics/2013/04/27/federal-warning-multiple-probes-follow-allegations-nevada-patient-dumping/

http://www.usatoday.com/story/news/nation/2013/04/17/nevada-buses-mentally-ill/2091727/

http://www.ktnv.com/news/local/204804721.html Here's a news story from a mother whose 18 year old son was given a bus pass and some medication from a hospital and sent on his way. He had been picked up walking barefoot down a highway. What's worse than the treatment by the hospital is the stupidity of the comments that follow. This is one of the biggest problems today and also the most frustrating. There are those that try to understand but just can't and then there are those that are just plain ignorant.

http://www.sacbee.com/leavinglasvegas/#storylink=misearch

NAMI

http://www.nami.org/Template.cfm?Section=Helpline1&template=/ContentManagement/ContentDisplay.cfm&ContentID=4859

Homelessness and the mentally ill

http://blogs.aljazeera.com/blog/americas/homelessness-rampant-among-us-mentally-ill

http://www.treatmentadvocacycenter.org/index.php?option=com_content&id=1379&Itemid=217

http://www.contracostatimes.com/ci_23148373/feds-must-probe-dumping-mentally-ill

Recognizing mental illness in the family

http://www.nmha.org/go/information/get-info/mi-and-the-family/recognizing-warning-signs-and-how-to-cope

How to help a loved one with mental illness

http://psychcentral.com/lib/15-ways-to-support-a-loved-one-with-serious-mental-illness/0007039

Hotlines

http://www.womenshealth.gov/mental-health/hotlines/

http://www.nami.org/Template.cfm?section=Find_Support

www.ingramcontent.com/pod-product-compliance
Lightning Source LLC
Chambersburg PA
CBHW081502170526
45166CB00008B/2516